Asthma in Focus

IN FOCUS series

The *In Focus* series is a group of introductory texts to the pharmaceutical care of patients with chronic conditions.

Pharmacy can play a large part in the management of chronic conditions and titles in the *In Focus* series provide practical information on the pharmaceutical care, medication and management of patients.

Each title includes an introduction to the condition; signs, symptoms and diagnosis; prevention and management; monitoring and treatment (including alternative treatments); care of the patient and the future.

Aimed at practising pharmacists in hospital and community, these introductory books will also be helpful to pre-registration and undergraduate pharmacy students, and healthcare professionals with an interest/working in the field of the specific chronic disease.

Available titles in the series:
Asthma in Focus, *Anna Murphy*
Schizophrenia in Focus, *David Taylor*
Diabetes in Focus, 2nd edition, *Anjana Patel*
Osteoporosis in Focus, *Niall Ferguson*
Parkinson's Disease in Focus, *Charles Tugwell*
Stroke in Focus, *Derek Taylor*

Asthma in Focus

Anna Murphy

MSc, MRPharmS

Consultant Respiratory Pharmacist
University Hospitals of Leicester NHS Trust, Leicester, UK

London • Chicago 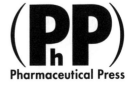 **Pharmaceutical Press**

2/07

Published by the Pharmaceutical Press
An imprint of RPS Publishing

1 Lambeth High Street, London SE1 7JN, UK
100 South Atkinson Road, Suite 200, Grayslake, IL 60030-7820, USA

© Pharmaceutical Press 2007

(**PP**) is a trademark of RPS Publishing

RPS Publishing is the publishing organisation of the Royal
Pharmaceutical Society of Great Britain

First published 2007

Typeset by Type Study, Scarborough, North Yorkshire
Printed in Great Britain by TJ International, Padstow, Cornwall

ISBN-10 0 85369 647 0
ISBN-13 978 0 85369 647 6

A catalogue record for this book is available from the British Library

Contents

Preface

There is currently no cure for asthma but available medication can control the inflammation, preventing symptoms and avoiding disability in the future from airway remodelling. Most patients with asthma can expect to live normal lives and have a normal life expectancy. However, asthma-related deaths and disability do still occur, often because patients don't have the appropriate medication or do not take their medication properly or regularly.

Good asthma care requires a team effort in both primary and secondary care. Following a diagnosis of asthma by a doctor, members of the team provide the patient with education and assess inhaler technique and day-to-day management of asthma. The management of medication is a specific role for pharmacists and they can help to drive improvements in patient outcomes. Pharmacists can also provide information and advice on lifestyle measures, an important component of total disease management.

A number of excellent and comprehensive books on asthma are available, although few are written with the pharmacist in mind. This book is intended to fill this gap. It is written for both specialist and non-specialist pharmacists working in all areas of the profession. It provides a general overview of asthma and covers subjects ranging from the basic mechanisms involved in asthma pathogenesis to patient-focused information on clinical management. In particular the book focuses on the medications available for asthma, how they work and when and how they should be used. The functional management approach to dealing with common clinical situations is based on the stepwise asthma management guideline developed by the British Thoracic Society and the Scottish Intercollegiate Guidelines Network (BTS/SIGN).

The BTS/SIGN published the new *British Guideline on the Management of Asthma* in February 2003. The guideline was based on a systematic review of the evidence, undertaken by multidisciplinary guideline development groups using SIGN methodology. It has always been recognised that if guidelines are to be used for the benefit of the patient, they must be kept up to date. The BTS/SIGN guideline is regularly updated to incorporate findings of the latest research and these updates are published on the BTS (www.brit-thoracic.org.uk) and SIGN (www.sign.ac.uk) websites. Insertions are marked with an arrow and year of the update. In April 2004, sections on pharmacological management, self-management and patient education, and the organisation and delivery of care for patients with asthma in primary care and hospital were updated. A further update in October 2005 reflected reviews of the sections on pharmacological management, inhaler devices, occupational asthma and audit and outcomes.

A major review, with publication of a revised paper copy of the guideline, is planned for early 2007.

In this book the original 2003 asthma management guideline is cited unless information has been updated, when the new reference is provided.

Recent changes in the National Health Service have made this an exciting time for the pharmacist, with opportunities for the pharmacist to enhance their role, providing services that have traditionally been carried out by doctors and nurses. The introduction of supplementary and independent prescribing, the new Community Pharmacy Contractual Framework and the new General Medical Service (GMS) contract all provide new opportunities for the pharmacy profession.

Details of supplementary prescribing by pharmacists were published in 2003. Supplementary prescribing is based on a prescribing partnership between an independent prescriber (i.e. a doctor or a dentist) and a supplementary prescriber. Supplementary prescribing can only be carried out within the previously agreed parameters of a patient-specific clinical management plan (CMP). This plan is drawn up, with the patient's agreement, following diagnosis by the independent prescriber and consultation and agreement between the independent and supplementary prescribers. It identifies the conditions to be treated and the circumstances under which the dosage, frequency and formulation of the medicines identified can be varied. The CMP relates to an individual patient and supplementary prescribing cannot take place without this document. Supplementary prescribing is useful for patients with on-going stable conditions, such as asthma, allowing the supplementary prescriber to deal with basic monitoring and repeat prescribing. Many pharmacists are embracing this extended role and are actively involved in the long-term management of patients with asthma and are providing medication review clinics.

From spring 2006, prescribing rights were extended to include independent prescribing for suitably trained pharmacists, meaning that they will be able to prescribe any licensed medicine for any medical condition within their individual area of competence, with the exception of controlled drugs. A pharmacist independent prescriber must accept full professional, clinical and medicolegal responsibility for their prescribing decisions. They should therefore only prescribe in situations where they feel fully competent, using medicines that they feel are effective for the patient and the condition being treated.

The new Community Pharmacy Contractual Framework will benefit patients with asthma by improving their access to healthcare advice and services. Under the new contract, community pharmacists can dispense repeat prescriptions, provide advice on healthy lifestyles and, in some cases, offer people with asthma and other chronic conditions a review of their medication.

The new GMS contact includes quality indicators for the management of asthma. These are evidence based and reflect a wide range of clinical, administrative and outcomes measures that will lead to improvement in the care of patients with asthma. The capacity issues within general practice and the increasing focus on chronic-disease management means that many GPs welcome the opportunity to direct patients to other healthcare professionals. The GMS contract provides opportunities for pharmacists to work alongside colleagues to improve asthma care, benefiting both the patient and the medical practice.

This book is designed to support the pharmacist in effective delivery of pharmaceutical care to patients with asthma. It also provides a useful reference tool for any health professional involved in the care of patients with asthma, particularly those with a prescribing role.

To encourage practical application of the information presented in this book, a series of 'Focus Points' are presented throughout the text. These 'Focus Points' provide summaries or overviews of key aspects of asthma management, which can be useful checklists in clinical practice.

While every effort has been made to ensure the accuracy of the information contained within the book, the rapidly changing nature of the subject matter must be borne in mind during its use. This is particularly important with respect to drug dosages and adverse effects. Pharmacists are advised to consult the most recent version of the manufacturer's summary of product characteristics (www.medicines. org.uk) or a current version of the *British National Formulary* to check dosage information.

It is intended that this book will aid all pharmacists involved with the care of patients with asthma to apply national and international guidelines on the treatment of asthma. I hope this book will be used to answer day-to day clinical problems in asthma management and will, in this way, support an individualised approach to treatment.

Anna Murphy
September 2006

Acknowledgements

I would like to thank my family and friends, particularly my husband Andrew, for their interest and encouragement throughout the preparation and writing of this book. The majority of this book was written during maternity leave after the birth of my twin daughters Lucy and Charlotte. I thank them for sleeping well and allowing me the time and energy to complete this. My sincere thanks are due to the staff at Pharmaceutical Press for their patience and for their input into the manuscript.

About the author

Anna Murphy is a consultant respiratory pharmacist at University Hospitals of Leicester NHS Trust and honorary senior lecturer at Leicester Warwick Medical School. She is also a national trainer for Education for Health (formerly the National Respiratory Training Centre). Anna led the development of the UK Clinical Pharmacy Association (UKCPA) Respiratory Practice Group and is currently chairperson.

Anna graduated in 1992 from Manchester University with a BSc(Hons) in Pharmacy, and completed her pre-registration training at The Royal Surrey County Hospital in Guildford, Surrey. Anna moved to Brighton where she worked for Brighton Healthcare from 1993 to 1997, gaining experience in all areas of hospital pharmacy and obtaining an MSc in Clinical Pharmacy from Brighton University. Leaving Brighton she moved to Leicester and was appointed as the Medicine and Respiratory Directorate Lead Pharmacist at Glenfield Hospital. In this post she developed the pharmaceutical service to the directorate, leading the Trust to support the novel role of a consultant pharmacist in respiratory medicine. Anna has undertaken this specialist post at The University Hospitals of Leicester NHS Trust since 2001.

Anna has also written chapters on medication management in pulmonary rehabilitation and a variety of articles on asthma, chronic obstructive pulmonary disease and chronic cough. She is currently developing her interest of concordance issues in patients with difficult asthma.

Focus points

Risk Factors Focus

Risk factors that increase the likelihood of the development of asthma   12
Triggers of asthma   19
Risk factors for near-fatal or fatal asthma   59
Causes of acute exacerbations of asthma   63
Factors that affect theophylline metabolism   206
Significant drug interactions with theophylline   211
Factors contributing to poor adherence to asthma treatment   244

Diagnostic Focus

Diagnosis of occupational asthma   15
Peak expiratory flow (PEF) measurements   21
Differential diagnoses of asthma   27
Comparison of asthma and chronic obstructive pulmonary disease (COPD)   28
Severity of acute asthma exacerbations and associated signs and symptoms in adults and children   65

Management Focus

Goals of asthma management   32
Dosages of inhaled corticosteroids equivalent to beclometasone, 200 micrograms/day   40
Immunosuppressive/corticosteroid-sparing therapy   46
Recommended interventions to reduce mortality and morbidity from asthma   60
Advice for avoiding house dust mites, from the BTS/SIGN asthma management guideline   83
Potential barriers to patient education   134
Sources of information for patients and healthcare professionals   136
Topics to be addressed with patients or parents/carers: the minimum information that should be provided to patients with asthma according to the asthma management guideline published by the BTS/SIGN   138
An example of an action plan for a patient with a personal-best PEF of 500 litres/minute   141

Inhalation Delivery Focus

Adverse Effects Focus

Monitoring Focus

1

Introduction

Asthma is a common chronic inflammatory disorder of the airways. Epidemiological studies indicate that asthma has become more common during the past two decades, especially among young children and in people living in urban areas. Between the early 1970s and the mid 1980s, prevalence increased by 50%.[1] This increase in asthma could be related to the fact that the prevalence of other atopic conditions, such as hay fever and eczema, also appears to be increasing.

Between 8 and 10% of children have been diagnosed with asthma, and approximately 5% of adults experience nocturnal breathlessness or have the reversible airflow limitation that defines asthma.[1] Overall, it has been estimated that 5.2 million people in the UK (1.1 million children and 4.1 million adults) are currently receiving treatment for asthma.[2] Worldwide, it is estimated that 300 million people now have asthma – striking evidence that asthma is a global health problem that cannot be ignored.

Asthma places a heavy burden on healthcare resources. Asthma costs the UK over £2.3 billion a year, an estimated £659 million of is in drug costs alone.[2] In addition, many working days are lost through sickness.

Asthma also leads to considerable morbidity and mortality. In England and Wales, there are approximately 100 000 hospital admissions for asthma annually.[1] Deaths from asthma in the UK peaked in the late 1980s at an annual rate of 39 deaths per million but had declined to 27 deaths per million by 1997. While this decrease is encouraging, too many patients still die as a consequence of asthma.

Asthma continues to have a major impact on patients' well-being and quality of life.[2-6] In the UK, 2.1 million people with asthma continue to experience symptoms regularly because they are not receiving appropriate care.[7] The Asthma Control and Expectations (ACE)[3] survey found that almost 70% of patients agreed with the statement, "I have to accept there are things I cannot do because of my asthma". Nearly half (46%) gave answers indicating that they did not feel well most of the time, and at least half reported symptoms on most days. The results of the ACE study supports those of the Asthma Insights and Reality in Europe (AIRE)[4] study, in which about 50% of patients considered their asthma to be well or completely controlled, despite reporting severe persistent symptoms. This survey found that 49% of respondents experienced activity limitation and 33% reported that their sleep had been affected by asthma. These results are similar to those obtained in the 1990/1991 National Asthma Survey and show that control of asthma has not changed in 10 years and is far from optimal.

The aims of asthma management are: the control of symptoms, including nocturnal symptoms and exercise-induced asthma, prevention of exacerbations, and the achievement of best possible pulmonary function, with minimal side-effects. Individual patients will have different goals and may wish to balance these aims against the potential side-effects or inconvenience of taking the medication necessary to achieve 'perfect' control. It is essential that each patient's treatment is individualised. The most recent published guidelines for the treatment of asthma are those produced by the British Thoracic Society (BTS) in collaboration with Scottish Intercollegiate Guidelines Network (SIGN).[8] The BTS/SIGN guideline adopts a 'stepwise' approach to treatment which aims to abolish symptoms as soon as possible and to optimise lung function by starting at a level of treatment that is most likely to achieve this; control is maintained by stepping up treatment as necessary and stepping it down when control is good. The pharmacological management plan is supported by avoidance of trigger factors as far as possible, patient education, concordance checks, instruction in inhaler technique and the development of a self-action plan for the patient.

The delivery of care to an asthmatic patient is a complex process. Poor control of asthma is often secondary to a number of factors. The medicines currently available to treat asthma are highly effective if prescribed and used correctly. However, it is estimated that metered-dose inhalers are used incorrectly by over 40% of people.[9,10] The choice of device may need to be individualised to ensure acceptability to the patient and effectiveness in practice. Patients often require reinforcement of technique by repeated advice and encouragement. This also may help to improve concordance rates. Health professionals may also have problems demonstrating inhaler technique and require training in order to teach patients correctly.[9]

Concordance with treatment regimens is a key issue in effective control of asthma. A recent analysis of data from UK asthma patients over 5 years revealed concordance rates estimated at 30% or less in 25% of patients.[11] Indeed, poor concordance with medication is believed to contribute to 18–48% of asthma-related deaths.[4] A host of factors is involved in poor concordance. It may reflect poor understanding by the patient of the benefits of treatment, inappropriate therapy and poor adherence to regular prophylactic therapy. Patients may not be able to afford prescription charges. Concordance with inhaled corticosteroids can be particularly problematic because, in contrast to short-acting bronchodilator therapy, patients are not immediately aware of the benefits of treatment; patients may also be worried about adverse effects. Educating the patient may help to allay their fears and improve concordance with medication. Providing patients with verbal and written information should enable them to take part in making decisions in managing treatment according to the level of symptoms.[12]

With good asthma care, patients experience fewer symptoms and improved quality of life, as well as fewer hospital admissions and fewer exacerbations. The responsibility for good asthma care lies with general practitioners, hospital doctors, specialist nurses and, increasingly, pharmacists. Every consultation with a patient with asthma is an opportunity to review, reinforce and extend both knowledge and skills.

References

1. National Asthma Campaign. Out in the open – a true picture of asthma in the United Kingdom today. *Asthma J* 2001; 6: 1–12.
2. Asthma UK. Where do we stand? Asthma in the UK today. Dec 2004. www.asthma.org.uk
3. Jones KG, Bell J, Fehrenbach C, *et al*. Understanding patient perceptions of asthma: results of the asthma control and expectations (ACE) survey. *Int J Clin Pract* 2002; 56: 89–93.
4. Rabe KF, Vermeire PA, Soriano JB, *et al*. Clinical management of asthma in 1999: the Asthma Insights and Realities in Europe (AIRE) study. *Eur Respir J* 2000; 16: 802–807.
5. Price D, Wolfe S. Delivery of asthma care: patients' use of and views on healthcare services, as determined from a nationwide interview survey. *Asthma J* 2000; 5: 141–144.
6. Smith NM. The 'Needs of People with Asthma' survey and initial presentation of the data. *Asthma J* 2000; 3: 133–144.
7. *Living on a knife edge: A powerful and moving account of living with serious symptoms of asthma*. Asthma UK, May 2004; www.asthma.org.uk.
8. British Thoracic Society, Scottish Intercollegiate Guidelines Network. British guideline on the management of asthma. *Thorax* 2003; 58 (Suppl I): S1–S94.
9. Tsang KW, Lam WK, Ip M, *et al*. Inability of physicians to use metered dose inhaler. *Asthma J* 1997; 34: 493–498.

10. Taylor D, Tunstell P. Metered dose inhaler: A system for assessing technique in patients and health professionals. *Pharm J* 1991; 246: 626–627.
11. Gupta RD, Guest JF. Factors affecting UK primary-care costs of managing patients with asthma over 6 years. *Pharmacoeconomics* 2003; 21: 357–369.
12. Partridge MR. Self-management in adults with asthma. *Patient Educ Counselling* 1997; 32: 1–4.

2

Asthma: the disease

Asthma-like symptoms were first recorded 3500 years ago in an Egyptian manuscript called *Ebers Papyrus*. Five hundred years later, the famous Greek physician Hippocrates first used the word asthma to describe an illness; the word means 'laboured breathing' in Greek. Until recently, asthma has been used to describe any disorder with episodic shortness of breath or dyspnoea, including 'cardiac asthma'; however, the definition has now been changed to exclude shortness of breath secondary to cardiac disease and relates only to a disorder of the respiratory system.

BTS/SIGN definition

The British Thoracic Society (BTS)/Scottish Intercollegiate Guidelines Network (SIGN) asthma management guideline[1] has adopted the definition of the International Consensus Report of 1992, which describes asthma as, 'a chronic inflammatory disorder of the airways which occurs in susceptible individuals; inflammatory symptoms are usually associated with widespread but variable airflow obstruction and an increase to a variety of stimuli. Obstruction is often reversible, either spontaneously or with treatment'.[2]

Important aspects that define asthma include airway hyper-responsiveness and bronchoconstriction.

Airway hyperresponsiveness

Hyperresponsiveness of the airways – a hallmark of clinical asthma[3] – refers to an increased tendency of the asthmatic airway to react to a variety of stimuli (triggers) that would not cause a response in a normal airway. These triggers can cause an asthma attack in an inflamed airway. For example, irritants such as smoke, dust, cold air and perfume can stimulate the airways and trigger an asthma attack. Studies have shown that the degree of bronchial hyperresponsiveness (BHR) correlates with the number of inflammatory cells recovered in bronchial alveolar fluid from the airways of asthmatic patients.[4] Clinically, the degree of BHR has been shown to correlate with general asthma severity, morning peak expiratory flow (PEF), the degree of diurnal variation of PEF and the frequency of inhaled beta-2-agonist use. The degree of BHR appears to decrease when asthma is well controlled with medication.[5]

Bronchoconstriction

Bronchoconstriction refers to a narrowing of the airways that causes obstruction of airflow (sometimes termed airflow limitation). This leads to the characteristic symptoms of asthma. The bronchoconstriction of asthma is unique because it is at least partly reversible, either spontaneously or with treatment. Inhalation of an allergen by a patient with allergic asthma causes prompt and significant bronchoconstriction. After this bronchial allergen challenge, there is a rapid decline in the patient's lung function, which usually begins within 15 minutes and generally subsides within the first hour (Figure 2.1). This immediate

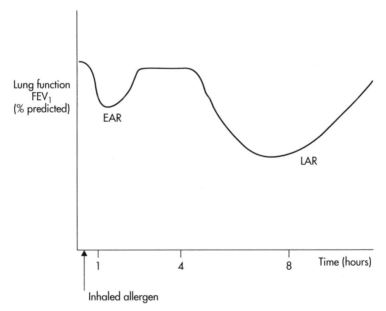

Figure 2.1   Changes in lung function (forced expiratory volume in 1 second; FEV_1) following inhalation of an allergen in an asthmatic patient, showing the classic early (EAR – Early Asthmatic Response) and late asthmatic responses (LAR – Late Asthmatic Response). (From Wardlaw AJ. *Asthma.* Oxford: BIOS Scientific Publishers Ltd, 1993. Reproduced with permission from the Taylor and Francis group.)

hypersensitivity has been termed an early asthmatic reaction or the early-phase response. After this initial phase, the airways return to a near-normal lung function either spontaneously or with the use of beta-2 agonists (e.g. salbutamol, terbutaline). However, in approximately 50% of patients, lung function will start to decline again after several hours. This late-phase response usually occurs 6–24 hours after exposure to the allergen and is termed the late asthmatic response. This late decline in lung function may be less severe than during the first response but is generally more prolonged, lasting several hours.[6]

Pathophysiology of the airway

The lumen of a normal airway has very little mucus present, allowing the free movement of air through the airway. A thin layer of mucus produced by the mucus gland protects the single layer of epithelial cells, which protect the bronchial wall. Infectious agents constantly enter the body via the respiratory system but several protective methods in the bronchi guard against these invaders so that, in a normal airway, the person will notice no changes to their breathing. These protective mechanisms are:

- recruitment of inflammatory cells from the bloodstream into the bronchial wall
- swelling of the bronchial wall and increased thickness of the airway smooth muscle
- mucus secretion
- constriction of the airway.

These processes are illustrated in Figure 2.2.

The histology changes significantly in the airways of an asthmatic patient. Post-mortem studies in patients who have died of asthma reveal the features of severe disease –grossly overinflated lungs, airways thickened by oedema and vasodilatation, spasm of hypertrophied smooth muscle and overproduction of mucus, with secretions forming plugs composed of cells and cellular debris. Histologically, plasma leaks from the blood vessels, contributing to both bronchial oedema and the eventual thickening of the bronchial wall. This thickening leads to chronic airway narrowing. Enlarged mucus glands secrete excess mucus and inflammatory cells, and inflammatory mediators enter the airway tissues and the lumen, causing an immune-mediated inflammation. Many cell-mediated immunological factors participate in the inflammatory

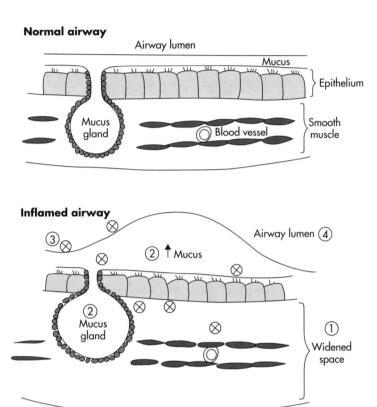

Figure 2.2 Schematic representation of the microscopic lung mucosa in a normal human airway and in an inflamed airway, illustrating the main cellular protective mechanisms: **1** increased airway smooth muscle thickness due to hyperplasia and/or hypertrophy; **2** goblet cell hyperplasia and increased mucus production; **3** recruitment of inflammatory mediators, mast cells, T lymphocytes and eosinophils into the airway tissue; **4** constriction of the airway.

process of asthma. The most important inflammatory cells involved are mast cells, T lymphocytes, macrophages and eosinophils. The inflammatory cells and mediators involved in the asthmatic inflammatory process are described in Table 2.1[7–9] and the relationships between the inflammatory mediators are shown in Figure 2.3.

Mast cells

Mast cell degranulation is important in the initiation of the immediate response following exposure to an allergen. Mast cells occur throughout

Table 2.1   The main inflammatory cells involved in the asthma process and the inflammatory mediators released by each

Inflammatory cell	Inflammatory mediators
Mast cells	Histamine, leukotrienes, proteases, pro-inflammatory cytokines (GM-CSF, interleukins), PAF, inflammatory factors of anaphylaxis
T lymphocytes	Pro-inflammatory cytokines
Macrophages and epithelial cells	Leukotrienes, pro-inflammatory cytokines, chemokines
Eosinophils	Leukotrienes, prostaglandins, granular proteins, pro-inflammatory cytokines, chemokines, PAF

GM-CSF, granulocyte monocyte colony stimulating factor; PAF, platelet activating factor.

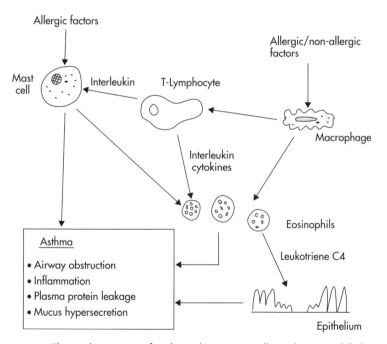

Figure 2.3   The pathogenesis of asthma: how mast cells and eosinophils become activated.

the walls of the respiratory tract and are found in increased numbers (3–5–fold) in the lungs of a patient with allergic asthma.[9] Mast cells bear receptors for immunoglobulin E (IgE) molecules on their surface, which bind IgE with high affinity. The bridging of adjacent IgE molecules by an allergen leads to the prompt release of mediators such as histamine, leukotrienes C4, D4 and E4, prostaglandins and platelet-activating factor from the mast cell. It is now known that mast cells also produce cytokines such as interleukin-4 (IL-4) and IL-5, which participate in allergic responses.[10] For example, IL-4 enhances IgE synthesis and IL-5 is essential for the formation and survival of eosinophils. There is also increasing evidence for the production of a number of other cytokines. Cytokines play an integral role in the coordination and persistence of the inflammatory process in chronic inflammation of the airways.[10]

T lymphocytes

T lymphocytes are responsible for much of the allergic inflammatory response in asthma. Following allergen presentation, T lymphocytes become activated and orchestrate the function of eosinophils and mast cells through the release of a number of interleukins.[9]

Macrophages

Macrophages are 'scavengers' in the airways, engulfing and digesting bacteria and other foreign material. A number of mediators produced and released by macrophages have been identified, such as platelet activating factor and leukotrienes B4, C4 and D4. Macrophages also produce chemicals that attract eosinophils to the area, which in turn facilitates inflammation.[9]

Eosinophils

Eosinophilia is a characteristic feature of all allergic diseases, including asthma, and is a feature of both atopic and non-atopic disease. Raised eosinophil counts are demonstrated in the airways of asthmatic patients, in the sputum or mucosal tissue. Eosinophils damage the airway epithelium and subsequently disrupt the normal physiology of the airways, contributing to the airway hyperresponsiveness characteristic of asthma.[11]

Airway remodelling

Airway remodelling can occur in the lung if the inflammation and bronchoconstriction are left untreated[12] and may be responsible for the chronic nature of asthma. It is thought that airway remodelling may be the cause of 'fixed' airflow obstruction in asthma that is not reversible with steroids or bronchodilators. Damage to the protective endothelial layer allows infiltration of inflammatory mediators into the mucosa. Hypertrophy of both muscle and mucus glands results in thicker secretions and bronchospasm (Figure 2.2).

These changes provide the rationale for the prompt and continued use of corticosteroids in asthma, as they effectively dampen down the inflammatory process in the lungs and prevent airway remodelling. Asthmatic patients should be aware of the long-term consequences of not taking regular inhaled corticosteroids.[12]

Risk factors

The risk factors for asthma can be divided into non-preventable and potentially preventable factors (see Risk Factors Focus, page 12). The non-preventable factors are important for identifying patients who are most at risk of developing asthma and could be used to identify patients in whom early intervention might be effective. The preventable risk factors, which are environmental in origin, may play a primary role in causing asthma or by precipitating or triggering asthma symptoms.

Clinical variants in asthma

Asthma has a number of clinical variants and, given the varied presentation and course of the disease, it is not surprising that asthma has been grouped in various ways. Traditionally, a fundamental division has been drawn between extrinsic (atopic) and intrinsic (non-atopic) asthma but there are also other classifications. These include types of asthma with specific trigger factors, such as occupational asthma, exercise-induced asthma, aspirin-sensitive asthma (ASA), allergic bronchopulmonary aspergillosis (ABPA) and asthma that is resistant to treatment with corticosteroids.

RISK FACTORS FOCUS

Risk factors that increase the likelihood of the development of asthma	
Non-preventable	
Sex	There is a clear sex difference in the prevalence of childhood asthma. Boys tend to predominate in the youngest age group; the sexes are equally represented at ages 12–14 years; girls predominate through the rest of the age range.
Family history	The likelihood of a child developing asthma is higher if one parent has asthma, with a risk of about 1 in 5, and even more likely if both parents have asthma, with a risk of about 2 out of 3 of developing asthma.
Season of birth	The season of birth affects age of first exposure to seasonal allergens. Generally, asthma is more prevalent in children born in the spring or summer.
Birth weight	Children who at birth were relatively heavy for their length have a slightly increased risk of developing asthma.
Family position and size	Asthma is more common in first born than in subsequent children.
Infection	Lack of contact with microorganisms and soil organisms may increase the incidence of asthma.
Low income	It is not clear whether the higher prevalence of asthma among this group is a function of other factors such as smoking, diet, residential status or work exposures.
Preventable	
Area of residence	Asthma is more common in rural than in urban setting and in inner cities than in suburbs.
Allergen exposure	Sensitisation to allergens (e.g. house dust mites, moulds, pollens, animals, cockroaches) early in life in genetically susceptible children may lead to the development of asthma.
Atmospheric pollution	Pollution has little or no effect on the prevalence of asthma, although it has a marked effect on the incidence of asthma exacerbations.
Environmental tobacco-smoke exposure	Fetal exposure to maternal smoking and exposure of infants and young children to second-hand smoke is a risk factor for asthma. The prevalence of asthma in children is about 25% higher in smoking than in non-smoking families. In adults, the effects of passive smoking on the prevalence of asthma is less dramatic but is still important.

continued overleaf

Risk Factors Focus (continued)	
Diet	There is some evidence that losing weight can relieve asthma symptoms. Breastfeeding may have a protective effect against asthma.
Physical activity and fitness	Obesity and physical inactivity are risk factors.
Immunisation	Some studies have suggested a link between the pertussis vaccination and a predisposition to asthma, but other studies have shown no effect.

Extrinsic versus intrinsic asthma

In many textbooks asthma is still classified as either extrinsic or intrinsic:

● extrinsic (atopic) – implying a definite cause
● intrinsic (or cryptogenic) – when no causative agent can be identified.

Extrinsic asthma occurs in atopic individuals who show positive skin-prick reactions to common inhaled allergens, the term 'extrinsic' basically meaning that an allergen from outside is thought to be the cause of the asthma. Asthma is more common in atopic individuals. Approximately 30% of the population make IgE against a variety of generally airborne antigens, such as faecal pellets from the house dust mite (*Dermatophagoides pteronyssinus*), grass pollen and cat and dog dander.[6] IgE binds tightly to receptors on the surface of the mast cell, which results in mast cell degranulation and the rapid release of histamine and other inflammatory mediators (Table 2.1). This is the classic type I hypersensitivity response.

Intrinsic asthma often starts in middle age. Many people with intrinsic asthma show positive skin-prick reactions and, on close questioning, give a history of respiratory symptoms compatible with childhood asthma.

In clinical practice, this classification is of little value. The distinction between these two types of asthma is largely academic, because many patients do not fit neatly into either category but instead have features of each. Non-atopic individuals may develop asthma in middle age from extrinsic causes such as sensitisation to occupational agents or aspirin intolerance or because they have taken beta-blockers. Extrinsic causes must be considered in all cases of asthma and avoided where possible.

Occupational asthma[1,13]

Asthma can also be triggered in the workplace. Asthma is described as 'work-related' when there is an association between symptoms and work. Work-related asthma has two distinct categories:

- *work-aggravated asthma* – pre-existing or coincidental new-onset adult asthma that is made worse by non-specific factors in the workplace
- *occupational asthma* – adult asthma caused by workplace exposure and not by factors outside of the workplace; it can occur in workers with or without previous asthma.

Occupational asthma can be further subdivided into:

- *allergic occupational asthma*, characterised by a latency period between first exposure to a trigger agent at work and the development of symptoms
- *irritant-induced occupational asthma*, which occurs typically within a few hours of a high-concentration exposure to an irritant gas, fume or vapour at work.

Occupational factors account for 9–15% of cases of asthma in adults of working age,[14] although the true incidence may in fact be higher, as many cases of occupational asthma remain undiagnosed. Diagnosis is based on a careful job history, detailed PEF recordings, including during work and rest periods (see Diagnostic Focus, page 15) and, if necessary, challenge with the suspected agent. Almost 90% of cases of occupational asthma are of the allergic type. Symptoms may resolve completely with early diagnosis and early removal from exposure, but for many patients asthma persists for several years after they are no longer exposed to the agent involved. In rare cases, occupational asthma has been fatal. The disease may leave people severely disabled, having to take early retirement, while many others have to change jobs to avoid contact with the substance that caused their asthma. Occupational asthma is unique in that it is the only type of asthma that is readily preventable. Prevention depends on the effective control or avoidance of the trigger agent and is the most important factor in reducing the impact of occupational asthma on individual workers and on society at large.

Exercise-induced asthma

Most patients with asthma experience an attack of wheezing after prolonged and continuous exercise. The symptoms of exercise-induced

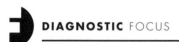

DIAGNOSTIC FOCUS

Diagnosis of occupational asthma[1]

Serial measurements of peak expiratory flow (PEF)

Measurements should be made every 2 hours from waking to sleeping for 4 weeks, keeping treatment constant and documenting times at work. Minimum standards for diagnostic sensitivity above 70% and specificity above 85% are:

- at least 3 days in each consecutive work period
- at least three series of consecutive days at work with three periods away from work (usually about 3 weeks)
- at least four evenly spaced readings per day.

This requires enthusiasm and attention to detail from the person with suspected occupational asthma. The aim is to see if occupational exposure provokes the asthma. Once occupational asthma has developed, the PEF will be influenced by waking time (often earlier on workdays), treatment and other provoking factors such as exercise and cold air. Once recorded, the PEF recordings need to be analysed by an expert and is best done with the aid of a criterion-based expert system (e.g. Oasys-2, which is a computer program that plots and interprets serial PEF readings of patients suspected as having occupational asthma). Suitable record forms and support are available from www.occupationalasthma.com.

---

asthma characteristically continue for some time after the exercise is completed rather than during the exercise period, the decrease in lung function reaching its maximum 5–20 minutes after stopping the activity. Symptoms often resolve spontaneously over the next 20–30 minutes. The mechanism proposed for exercise-induced asthma is that the hyperventilation of exercise results in cooling and drying of the airways, which subsequently causes mediator release and bronchospasm. In spite of the fact that physical exercise adversely affects patients with asthma, patients should not be discouraged from participating. Serious athletes can change their training programme and competition pattern to limit the effects of the exercise-induced asthma.

The diagnosis of exercise-induced asthma is usually made on the basis of patient's history. If the history is unclear, however, an exercise challenge test can be used to establish the diagnosis. A 15% or greater decrease in PEF or forced expiratory flow in 1 second (FEV$_1$; the maximum volume of air expired in 1 second from full inspiration) (measured just before and then at 5 minute intervals after exercise for 30–60 minutes) is good documentation of exercise-induced asthma.

For most people with asthma, exercise-induced asthma is an expression of poorly controlled asthma; regular treatment including inhaled steroids should therefore be reviewed.[1]

Aspirin-sensitive asthma

Most patients with asthma can take aspirin or other non-steroidal anti-inflammatory drugs (NSAIDs) with no problem. However, up to 10% of patients with chronic asthma are intolerant of aspirin and its ingestion can induce acute bronchoconstriction, profuse rhinorrhoea, facial flushing and, in severe cases, anaphylaxis and even death.[15] These symptoms can occur within minutes or hours. It has been estimated that up to 25% of hospital admissions for asthma that require mechanical ventilation could be the result of NSAID ingestion.[16] About half of patients with ASA have more severe asthma, and a significant proportion require regular oral corticosteroids to control symptoms. ASA is often associated with recurrent nasal polyps and rhinosinusitis with prominent nasal congestion and a loss of smell and taste.

Aspirin blocks the production of prostaglandins by inhibiting the action of cyclo-oxygenase (COX). Some prostaglandins are pro-inflammatory mediators, supporting the use of aspirin to treat inflammatory conditions such as rheumatoid arthritis, whereas other prostaglandins are anti-inflammatory. PG_{E2} is a COX product of airway epithelium and smooth muscle, and is considered to be immunodulatory and predominately bronchoprotective. *In vitro* studies have shown that PG_{E2} inhibits many inflammatory events, including release of mediators from mast cells and eosinophil activation.[17] Inhibition of COX prevents the anti-inflammatory action of prostaglandin PG_{E2}. and also leads to increased production of the leukotrienes, because the breakdown of arachidonic acid is redirected via the alternative 5-lipoxygenase route to the leukotrienes (Figure 2.4). Leukotrienes are potent inflammatory mediators that cause bronchoconstriction, mucus hypersecretion, vasopermeability and airway hyperresponsiveness in patients with asthma. They exert their effects by binding to the cysteinyl leukotriene receptor. Leukotriene receptor antagonists (e.g. montelukast and zafirlukast) reduce asthma symptoms induced by an aspirin challenge in patients with ASA. Symptoms of ASA can also be reduced by desensitisation with incremental doses of oral aspirin. In general, any NSAID that blocks the cyclo-oxygenase pathway induces similar symptoms in any patient with

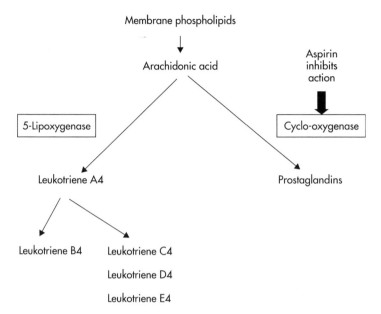

Figure 2.4 Biosynthetic pathways leading to the production of leukotrienes and prostaglandins.

ASA. Patients with ASA must therefore avoid aspirin and other NSAIDs.[18,19]

Allergic bronchopulmonary aspergillosis

The incidence of allergic bronchopulmonary aspergillosis (ABPA) is estimated to be 1% in asthmatics but the exact figure is unknown. ABPA is characterised by asthma, peripheral blood eosinophilia and transient shadows on chest radiograph. It results from an allergic reaction to *Aspergillus fumigatus*, a fungus that colonises the airway. Early on, the allergic response causes bronchoconstriction, but permanent damage occurs as the inflammation persists, causing bronchiectasis. ABPA is diagnosed if asthma is present together with shadows on the chest radiograph, a raised serum IgE concentration and presence of IgG precipitating antibodies, a raised eosinophil count and *A. fumigatus* cultured in the sputum. It is almost impossible to eradicate the fungus, although the azole antifungal drugs may be helpful in controlling ABPA. High-dose oral corticosteroids are given to reduce the inflammation. It is not known why some asthmatics develop ABPA.

Corticosteroid-resistant asthma

Corticosteroids are the mainstay of treatment for patients with asthma by virtue of their anti-inflammatory properties (see Chapter 12). In over 90% of patients with asthma, a dose of corticosteroid results in an improvement in PEF readings by more than 20%. However, 1–5% of patients with asthma, who tend to be at the more severe end of the disease spectrum, show no improvement in symptoms or lung function. The reason for this is unknown.

Diagnosis of asthma

A careful medical history, physical examination and lung function tests provide the information needed to diagnose most cases of asthma. However, diagnosis is not always straightforward and it can take time to make an accurate diagnosis. Eczema, hay fever and a family history of asthma or atopic diseases are often associated with asthma but they are not necessarily elements of an asthma diagnosis. There is no single satisfactory diagnostic test for all asthma.

Medical history

Patients with asthma typically present repeatedly to their doctor with respiratory problems. The frequency and duration of attacks varies tremendously from patient to patient and in the same patient over time.

The usual presenting features of asthma are:

- wheeze
- shortness of breath
- chest tightness
- cough, particularly at night and early in the morning.

Wheezing is caused by airflow limitation, resulting in a high-pitched whistling sound that is usually heard on expiration but may also be heard on inspiration. Chest tightness or dyspnoea is the sensation that patients often feel in association with the increased work needed to breathe when the airways are constricted. Cough probably results from stimulation of sensory nerves in the airways by inflammatory mediators that are released by various inflammatory cells involved in asthma.

Other symptoms include:

- difficulty in sleeping
- chest pain
- vomiting
- itching (usually in children).

Symptoms tend to be variable, intermittent, worse at night and are provoked by triggers (see Risk Factors Focus, below). It is important to know the age at which the first attack occurred and the pattern of symptoms, whether they are continuous or episodic, have a seasonal or perennial appearance or day–night variation, whether they worsen indoors or outdoors, at home or in the work place. Information that provides indications of or clues to asthma severity are the number of nights per month with asthma symptoms, the frequency of broncho-dilator use and limitation of physical activities. For patients whose asthma is more severe, it is important to ascertain the number of times the patient is admitted to hospital because of their asthma. The onset, duration and frequency of symptoms should be carefully investigated in addition to their type and severity.

RISK FACTORS FOCUS

Triggers of asthma

- Hyperventilation
- Drugs – aspirin, non-steroidal anti-inflammatory drugs, muscle relaxants (e.g. suxamethonium, atracurium), parasympathomimetics (e.g. pilocarpine, carbachol) and beta-blockers. Non-selective beta-blockers such as propranolol can trigger severe asthma and even cardioselective ones such as atenolol and bisoprolol may provoke bronchospasm.
- House dust mite
- Foods and drinks, such as nuts, milk and eggs
- Pollens
- Preservatives (e.g. metabisulfite) or colouring agents (e.g. tartrazine)
- Animal danders
- Gastro-oesophageal reflux
- Occupational agents
- Environmental pollutants (e.g. traffic fumes) or irritants (e.g. cigarette smoke)
- Exercise
- Common viral infections of the upper respiratory tract
- Cold air
- Aerosols

Physical examination

Although a physical examination is an important diagnostic tool in establishing the severity of an exacerbation, it is of little help in the diagnosis of intermittent and mild asthma when bronchial obstruction is either absent or mild. However, if signs of airflow obstruction are present at the time of the examination, analysis of these signs can give an accurate picture of the severity of asthma. As mentioned above, expiratory wheeze is the most typical sign of asthma. It provides a guide to severity but it should not be forgotten that expiratory wheeze may be absent in a severe asthma exacerbation, when the patient is too weak to generate enough airflow turbulence in their much narrowed airways. Other signs of worsening asthma include inability to speak in complete sentences, hyperinflated chest, the use of accessory muscles of respiration with intercostal recession, cyanosis, pulsus paradoxus of greater than 15 mmHg, hyperresonance of percussion note and drowsiness. Occasionally, in acute severe asthma, there may be evidence of lobar collapse caused by mucus plugging of the large airways.

Objective diagnostic measurements

Measurement of the patient's lung function is useful both for diagnosis of asthma and to monitor the course of the disease (see Chapter 6). Such tests include spirometry, which provides an assessment of airflow limitation, and PEF, which measures the maximum speed at which air can flow out of the lungs. Asthma is an obstructive lung disease, characterised by a decrease in PEF and FEV_1, although these may be normal if measured between episodes of bronchospasm. If they are repeatedly normal in the presence of symptoms, then a diagnosis of asthma is doubtful.

Peak expiratory flow measurements

PEF is the highest flow obtained during a forced expiration starting immediately after a deep inspiration at total lung capacity. It is a reproducible index and can be measured with inexpensive, simple-to-use, portable peak flow meters. Home monitoring of the patient's PEF over a 2-week period can help with the diagnosis of asthma, which is based on the demonstration of diurnal variability in PEF of greater than 20%, with a minimal change of at least 60 L/minute, ideally for 3 days in a week for 2 weeks seen over a period of time.[1] The percentage variability is calculated by recording the highest and lowest peak flow measurements during the day (see Diagnostic Focus, page 21).

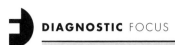

DIAGNOSTIC FOCUS

Peak expiratory flow (PEF) measurements

Amplitude = highest PEF − lowest PEF

$$\% \text{ PEF variability} = \frac{\text{highest PEF} - \text{lowest PEF}}{\text{highest PEF}} \times 100$$

Example
Highest PEF = 500 L/minute
Lowest PEF = 350 L/minute
Amplitude = 500 − 350 = 150 L/minute

$$\% \text{ PEF variability} = \frac{150}{500} \times 100 = 30\%$$

This example shows a 30% change in variability throughout the day with a 150 L/minute change.

Both values are above the diagnostic threshold of 20% and 60 L/minute, respectively, suggesting asthma as a possible diagnosis.

Spirometry

The patient's lung function and expiratory flows can be measured using a spirometer, which is the gold standard in the diagnosis and monitoring of asthma severity. Spirometry is recommended in the initial assessment of all patients with suspected asthma but not all primary care practices have access to a spirometer. Measurements useful for the diagnosis of asthma include the forced vital capacity (FVC; the maximum volume of air that can be exhaled from the lung), FEV_1 and the FEV_1/FVC ratio. Spirometry is helpful in making the initial diagnosis in a patient presenting with breathlessness, as it can help distinguish between obstructive and restrictive lung disease.

- In an obstructive disease in which the airways are narrowed (e.g. asthma, chronic obstructive pulmonary disease (COPD) or cystic fibrosis), FEV_1 is predominately reduced and the FVC is normal or only slightly reduced, making the FEV_1/FVC ratio lower than normal (i.e. a ratio of less than 80%).
- In a restrictive lung disorder (e.g. fibrosing alveolitis or malignant infiltration), the FVC and FEV_1 are both reduced to a greater extent and the FEV_1/FVC ratio is usually higher than normal (i.e. over 80%).

A diagnosis of asthma, demonstrating the reversibility component of the disease, can be shown by an increase in the patient's lung function after either a single inhalation of a short-acting beta-2 agonist (e.g. salbutamol, 400 micrograms by metered-dose inhaler and a spacer device or 2.5 mg by nebuliser) or a trial of steroid tablets (e.g. prednisolone, 30 mg daily for 14 days).

Each of these methods can be used, measuring either PEF (20% change from baseline and at least 60 L/minute) or FEV_1 (15% change and at least 200 mL). Further information on lung function tests is provided in Chapter 6.

Bronchial hyperresponsiveness

As mentioned above, the airways of patients with asthma demonstrate BHR, which is the increased bronchoconstrictor response to a variety of physical, chemical and pharmacological stimuli. Changes in the patient's lung function (usually FEV_1) is measured after inhalation of incremental doses of a stimulant (e.g. histamine or methacholine).[3] The airway response develops at lower levels of stimulation in patients with asthma and the intensity of BHR is more severe. BHR is described in terms of the concentration of either methacholine or histamine that causes a 20% reduction in the patient's lung function (FEV_1), known as the Pc20. The Pc20 of a random population is normally distributed, patients with asthma being clustered to the left of the curve (see Figure 2.5). A Pc20 of less than 4 mg/mL methacholine is highly suggestive of asthma.[20] This is a useful test in patients in whom the diagnosis of asthma is uncertain. It is also an objective measure of asthma severity.

In children, exercise provocation is usually preferred as it is a more natural stimulation and children often tolerate it better.

Exercise tests

Exercise tests are widely used in the diagnosis of asthma, mainly in children. Lung function (either PEF or FEV_1) is measured at rest, after 6 minutes of exercise (e.g. running) and then every 10 minutes for 30 minutes. A decrease in lung function – 20% change in PEF from baseline and at least 60 L/minute) or 15% change in FEV_1 from baseline and at least 200 mL – suggests a diagnosis of asthma, although a negative test does not rule out this diagnosis. As this procedure may occasionally induce significant asthma, facilities for immediate treatment should be available.

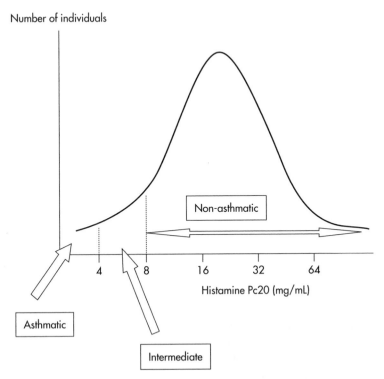

Number of individuals

Non-asthmatic

Asthmatic

Intermediate

4   8   16   32   64

Histamine Pc20 (mg/mL)

Figure 2.5   Distribution of histamine Pc20 values (the concentration of histamine required to cause a 20% decrease in lung function, forced expiratory volume in 1 second) in the general population.[15]
Source: Wardlaw, A.J. *Distribution of histamine Pc20 values in the general population, Asthma*, p.g.[6]

Blood and sputum tests

Investigations for atopy, such as measurement of serum IgE concentration and sputum and blood eosinophil counts, are not necessary to make the diagnosis of asthma, but may help differentiate asthma from COPD in adults. Patients with asthma, particularly during an exacerbation, may show an increase in the number of eosinophils in peripheral blood ($>0.4 \times 10^9$/L).[21] This shows the presence of inflammation but not the severity of airway inflammation. Very high peripheral blood eosinophil counts may indicate a diagnosis of aspergillosis or other hyper-eosinophilic syndromes.

Cell counts of induced sputum from normal individuals show a predominance of macrophages and neutrophils, with only an occasional eosinophil whereas in adults and children with asthma there is an increase in the proportion and number of eosinophils. The degree of sputum eosinophilia is higher in symptomatic asthma than in patients with well-controlled asthma. Thus, sputum eosinophilia may reflect disease activity, and may help in the assessment of severity. In addition, sputum eosinophilia is usually associated with a poor response to or non-compliance with corticosteroids.

Induction of sputum by inhalation of hypertonic sodium chloride has proved to be a reliable and safe method for analysing inflammatory cells from the major airways of patients. Occasionally, broncho-constriction can occur, so patients should be monitored carefully throughout the procedure. Bronchoconstriction can be reduced by pre-treatment with a beta-2 agonist, which does not alter the cellular differential.[22]

Nitric oxide in exhaled air

Nitric oxide (NO) is considered to be a biochemical indicator of the function of airways. It is formed by cells in the lungs and plays a key role in the regulation of a wide variety of pulmonary functions. NO acts as a vasodilator and bronchodilator and is an important mediator of the inflammatory process. Exhaled NO is increased in asthma, and levels are altered by treatment with anti-inflammatory therapy.[23] Monitoring of NO can be done by exhaling into a chemiluminescence analyser, making it an attractive test to highlight the presence of airway inflam-mation and for monitoring asthma control. Studies have shown that the exhaled NO concentration is higher in steroid-naive subjects with asthma than in normal subjects, and in atopic compared with non-atopic normal subjects. Exhaled NO levels increase when control of asthma deteriorates and when asthma is exacerbated.[24] However, many other factors can affect the level of exhaled NO, and levels are increased in several diseases other than asthma, such as upper and lower respiratory tract infections, pulmonary tuberculosis and in bronchiectasis. Decreased NO levels are seen after inhaled or oral corticosteroids, smoking, acute alcohol ingestion in asthmatics and in patients with cystic fibrosis, COPD or heart failure. These observations suggest that the clinical measurement of exhaled NO is limited and will not be useful in monitoring the control or diagnosis of asthma.

Chest radiograph

There are no diagnostic features of asthma on the chest radiograph although hyperinflation of the lungs may be observed in acute exacerbations. A chest radiograph may be useful in excluding differential diagnoses such as pneumothorax. Chest radiographs should be performed in any patient with atypical symptoms.

Skin-prick tests

Skin-prick testing is of no value in diagnosing asthma (although they may be useful in identifying triggers) but are first choice in the diagnosis of allergy. Skin-prick test are simple, easy and rapid to perform and are highly sensitive and specific. Many patients with asthma are atopic, and their reaction to a wide range of external allergens can be a common exacerbating factor of asthma. When performing a skin-prick test, a drop of each allergen solution is distributed on the forearm and a needle introduced through the drop into the skin surface to a depth of about 1 mm. The patient's skin reaction at the site, if any, is assessed 15–20 minutes later. A positive wheal-and-flare reaction indicates that specific IgE antibodies to that particular allergen are bound to mast cells in the skin. Skin-prick tests are reproducible and seldom produce systemic reactions.

Diagnosis in children

Epidemiological studies suggest that asthma in children in particular is often underdiagnosed or misdiagnosed. However, diagnosis of asthma in young children can be difficult. Asthma should be suspected in any child with wheezing, but not all wheeze is due to asthma. In children under 5 years of age, the most common cause of asthmatic symptoms (i.e. wheezing and cough) is a viral upper respiratory tract infection.

Two general patterns of wheezing are seen in young children.

- The first, which is also the most frequent pattern, is a self-limiting condition in which there is an eventual resolution of wheezing during the preschool years (less than 5 years of age), possibly as a result of airway growth. The majority of children who wheeze in the first few years of life will no longer be wheezing by school age (approximately 5 years of age). They may not need aggressive treatment as they may be more at risk from the effects of the medication than the disease.
- The second pattern is continued wheezing throughout childhood. Persistent wheeze has strong associated risk factors, such as atopy (e.g. eczema, rhinitis and food allergy), a family history of atopy (allergy or asthma) and perinatal exposure to passive smoke or inhaled allergens. Asthma is linked to both parental and sibling atopy but the strongest association is with maternal atopy. A maternal history of asthma or atopy is a

significant risk factor for late-onset childhood asthma and recurrent wheezing throughout childhood.

The presence of allergy is not essential to the diagnosis of asthma, but its absence in a schoolchild with symptoms suggestive of asthma should prompt consideration of alternative diagnoses. In schoolchildren, the diagnosis can be confirmed by bronchodilator responsiveness, PEF variability or tests of BHR. The diagnosis of asthma in children should therefore be based on the following:[1]

- the presence of key features and careful consideration of alternative diagnoses
- assessment of the response to trials of treatment and ongoing assessment
- repeated reassessment of the child, questioning the diagnosis if management is ineffective.

Diagnosis in the elderly

Asthma is common in the elderly but a life of exposure to smoking or inhaled environmental irritants makes COPD a more frequent differential diagnosis. Proper diagnosis in these patients can be complicated by the difficulty some older people have in performing lung function tests. However, it is important to determine the extent of reversibility of airflow obstruction. If reversibility can be demonstrated, the patient should receive appropriate management for asthma. If asthma is present, it tends to be severe, with a proneness to exacerbations, possibly because of underdiagnosis, undertreatment or poor perception of symptoms. Occasionally, asthma can be associated with the use of medications such as NSAIDS or beta-blockers. Drugs that induce or aggravate asthma should be withdrawn if possible.

Differential diagnosis

Several conditions should be considered in the differential diagnosis of asthma. These conditions vary significantly depending on the patient's age. All differential diagnoses should be excluded (see Diagnostic Focus, page 27).

Children

In infants with a suspected diagnosis of asthma, congenital malformations (e.g. tracheo-oesophageal fistula, vascular rings) should be considered and appropriate evaluations performed to rule out such

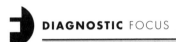

Differential diagnoses of asthma

Chronic obstructive pulmonary disease
Cardiac disease
Tumour (laryngeal, tracheal, lung)
Bronchiectasis
Foreign body
Interstitial lung disease
Pulmonary embolus
Aspiration
Vocal cord dysfunction
Hyperventilation
Eosinophilic pneumonitis (Churg–Strauss syndrome)
Psychological factors

malformations. Young children commonly have viral upper respiratory tract infections that can cause symptoms similar to those of an asthma exacerbation. Obstruction with a foreign body must be considered in children who have rapid onset of unilateral wheezing. Underlying disorders such as cystic fibrosis and immunodeficiency disease should be considered in children with chronic cough and sputum production.

Adults

Heart failure and COPD are the primary diseases that need to be considered in the differential diagnosis of asthma in adults. Less commonly, patients with obstruction of the large airways, whether from tumours, vocal cord dysfunction or sarcoidosis present with wheezing.

COPD versus asthma

Differentiating between asthma and COPD can be difficult, as these diseases share bronchial obstruction as a common symptom and may produce similar changes in lung function. Both diseases are chronic, produce persistent inflammatory changes in the airways (pathologically, the inflammation differs slightly in the two conditions: eosinophils predominate in asthma whereas neutrophils predominate in COPD) and airflow obstruction. However, the underlying disease processes are different and require different management and treatment. Patients with

COPD are treated as asthmatics far too often. Failure to distinguish between asthma and COPD in older patients can lead to inappropriate and ineffective treatment. The Diagnostic Focus below summarises the differences between COPD and asthma in terms of causative factors and the ability of the airways to return to normal.[25]

DIAGNOSTIC FOCUS

Comparison of asthma and chronic obstructive pulmonary disease (COPD)[24]		
	Asthma	**COPD**
Age at onset	Any, but most likely below 40 years	Mainly 50 years and higher
Smoking history	+/–	++
Family history of atopy/asthma	++	+/–
Presence of hay fever or eczema	++	+/–
Intermittent symptoms brought on by trigger symptoms	++	–
Nocturnal symptoms	++	+/–
Symptoms constant	–	++
Symptoms progressive	+	++
PEF variable	++	–
Responsive to bronchodilator	++	+/–
Responsive to corticosteroid	++	+/–

PEF, peak expiratory flow.

References

1. British Thoracic Society/Scottish Intercollegiate Guidelines Network. British guideline on the management of asthma. *Thorax* 2003; 58 (Suppl I) S1–S94.
2. International consensus report on the diagnosis and treatment of asthma. Bethesda, Maryland: National Heart, Lung and Blood Institute, National Institutes of Health 20892. Publication no. 92–3091, March 1992. *Eur Respir J* 1992; 5: 601–641.
3. Cockcroft DW, Killian DN, Mellon JJ, *et al*. Bronchial reactivity to inhaled histamine: a method and clinical survey. *Clin Allergy* 1977; 7: 235–243.
4. Murray JF, Nadel JA, eds. *Textbook of Respiratory Medicine Vol. 1*, 3rd edn. Philadelphia: WB Saunders, 2000.
5. Juniper EF, Frith PA, Hargreave FE. Airway responsiveness to histamine and methacholine: relationship to minimum treatment to control symptoms of asthma. *Thorax* 1981; 36: 575–579.

6. Wardlaw AJ. *Asthma*. Oxford: BIOS Scientific Publishers Ltd, 1993.
7. Barnes PJ, Chung KF, Page CP. Inflammatory mediators of asthma: an update. *Pharmacol Rev* 1998; 50: 515–596.
8. Bousquet J, Jeffery PK, Busse WW, *et al*. Asthma. From bronchoconstriction to airways inflammation and remodelling. *Am J Respir Care Med* 2000; 161: 1720–1745.
9. Djukanovic R, Holgate ST. *An Atlas of Asthma*. Carnforth UK: Parthenon Publishing, 1999.
10. Chung KF, Barnes, PJ. Cytokines in asthma. *Thorax* 1999; 54: 825–857.
11. Rothenberg ME. Eosinophilia. *N Engl J Med* 1998; 338: 1592–1600.
12. Redington AE, Howarth PH. Airway wall remodelling in asthma (editorial). *Thorax* 1997; 52: 310–312.
13. British Occupational Health Research Foundation (BOHRF). *Occupational Asthma. Identification, Management and Prevention: Evidence Based Review and Guidelines*, 2004. http: //www.bohrf.org.uk/content/asthma.htm
14. Meredith S, Nordman H. Occupational asthma: measures of frequency from four countries. *Thorax* 1996; 51: 435–440.
15. Knox A. How prevalent is aspirin induced asthma? *Thorax* 2002; 57: 565.
16. Marquette CH, Saulnier F, Leroy O. Long term prognosis of near fatal asthma: a 6 year follow up study of 145 asthmatic patients who underwent mechanical ventilation for a near-fatal attack of asthma. *Am Rev Respir Dis* 1992; 146: 76–81.
17. Koshkas K, Papatheodorou G, Psathakis K *et al*. Prostaglandin E2 in the expired breath condensate of patients with asthma. *Eur Respir J* 2003; 22: 743–747.
18. Szczeklik A, Niżankowska E. Clinical features and diagnosis of aspirin induced asthma. *Thorax* 2000; 55 (Suppl 2): S42–S44.
19. Schiavino D, Nucera E, Milani A, *et al*. The aspirin disease. *Thorax* 2000; 55 (Suppl 2): S66–S69.
20. Cockcroft DW, Berscheid BA, Murdock KY. Unimodel distribution of bronchial responsiveness to inhaled histamine in a random human population. *Chest* 1983; 83: 751.
21. Bousquet J, Chanez P, Lacoste JY, *et al*. Eosinophilic inflammation in asthma. *N Engl J Med* 1990; 323: 1033–1039.
22. Hargreave FE. Induced sputum for the investigation of airway inflammation. *Can Respir J* 1999; 6: 169–174.
23. Kharitonov SA, Yates D, Robbins RA, *et al*. Increased nitric oxide in exhaled air of asthmatic patients. *Lancet* 1994; 343 (8890): 133–135.
24. Massaro AF, Gaston B, Kita D, *et al*. Expired nitric oxide levels during treatment of acute asthma. *Am J Respir Crit Care Med* 1995; 152: 800–803.
25. British Thoracic Society. BTS Guidelines for the management of chronic obstructive pulmonary disease. *Thorax* 1997; 52 (Suppl 5): S1–S28.

3

Pharmacological management

Aims of pharmacological management

The main aims in the treatment of chronic asthma are to control the disease and to prevent irreversible airway damage and mortality from asthma (see Management Focus, page 32). Control of the disease is usually defined as:[1]

- minimal symptoms during the day and night
- no exacerbations
- minimal need for rescue/reliever medication
- normal levels of activity, including during exercise and sports
- normal lung function (forced expiratory volume in 1 second [FEV_1] or peak expiratory flow (PEF) greater than 80% predicted or best)
- minimal adverse effects from the anti-asthma treatment.

Control of asthma can be achieved in the majority of patients using currently available medications, although complete control may not be possible for some patients, especially those with severe disease, either because the dosages of medication required for 'perfect control' produce unacceptable adverse effects for the patient or because the patient is not prepared to follow the therapeutic recommendations completely. Individual patients will have different expectations of treatment from the health professional, and a compromise may have to be reached in order to achieve the best achievable control of symptoms. Treatment goals are best met by discussing treatment plans with the patient, and by primary and secondary care working together. Communication between all involved is the key to successful management.

Asthma is a complex disease and it is essential that each patient's treatment is individualised. The treatment plan should take into account the disease severity, the patient's environment and exercise levels, any concordance problems, the patient's understanding of both the disease

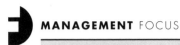

Goals of asthma management

- Minimise or eliminate symptoms
- Maximise lung function
- Prevent exacerbations
- Minimise the need for medication
- Minimise side-effects of treatment
- Provide enough information and support to facilitate self-management
- Promote patient concordance with medication regimen
- Maintain normal growth (children)

and the treatment and their ability to use an inhaler device. The main aim should be to provide patients with the skills they need to manage and control the disease for themselves.

Pharmacological treatment

The treatment of asthma has changed drastically since this advice published in the *Illustrated Doctor* in 1934: "The treatment during an attack is to provide the patient with as much fresh air as possible and to let him choose the position in which he feels easiest. If the attack follows a heavy meal his sufferings may be shortened by an emetic composed of mustard in water. A cup of strong coffee is often found beneficial during attacks, or a capsule of amyl nitrate may be broken and inhaled."[2]

Understanding of the pathophysiology of asthma has led to the development of medications to treat and prevent acute episodes. For many years, the aim of treatment was to control an acute attack. More recently, however, with the recognition that asthma is a chronic condition rather than an episodic disease, the focus of therapy has shifted to long-term control with medications that may alter the course of the disease. Effective treatments should suppress inflammation over the long term and prevent exacerbations; hence, inhaled corticosteroids (ICS) are the cornerstone of long-term therapy.

Pharmacological therapy is used to prevent and control asthma symptoms, reduce the frequency and severity of asthma exacerbations and reverse airflow obstruction. Medications for asthma are divided into two general classes.

- *Preventer medications* are taken daily on a long-term basis to achieve and maintain control of persistent asthma (these medications are also known as long-term controllers).
- *Quick reliever medications* are taken to provide prompt reversal of acute airflow obstruction and relief of bronchoconstriction (these medications are also known as relief or rescue medications).

The majority of patients with persistent asthma require both classes of medication. However, optimal control is achieved when no or little quick reliever medication is needed. The individual drugs used to treat asthma are discussed in Chapters 10–14.

Preventer medications

Long-term controller or preventer medications are usually prescribed for use on a daily basis, with the aim to achieve and maintain control of persistent asthma. They include corticosteroids (anti-inflammatory), long-acting bronchodilators and leukotriene receptor antagonists (see Chapters 10, 12 and 14). The corticosteroids are the most effective in controlling the disease, reducing the markers of airway inflammation (e.g. eosinophils) within the mucosa of the airway and thus decreasing the intensity of airway hyperresponsiveness.

Quick reliever medications

Quick reliever medications are used to provide prompt relief of bronchoconstriction and its accompanying acute symptoms (cough, chest tightness and wheezing). They do not contribute substantially to the long-term control of asthma. In fact, frequent or regular use of quick reliever medications may even decrease long-term control of asthma either by decreasing concordance with long-term preventer medication or by mechanisms not yet fully understood.[3] Quick reliever medications include short-acting beta-2 agonists (SABAs), anticholinergics, quick-acting methylxanthine preparations and short courses of corticosteroids (see Chapters 10, 11 and 13). Although the onset of action is slow (>4 hours), short courses of systemic corticosteroids are important in the treatment of moderate-to-severe exacerbations because they prevent progression of the exacerbation, speed recovery and prevent early relapses.

Management of chronic asthma

The British Thoracic Society (BTS) has collaborated with the Scottish Intercollegiate Guidelines Network (SIGN) to publish guidance on the management of asthma.[1] The guideline recommends a stepwise approach to the treatment of chronic asthma, illustrated in Figure 3.1 (adults), Figure 3.2 (children aged 5–12 years) and Figure 3.3 (children

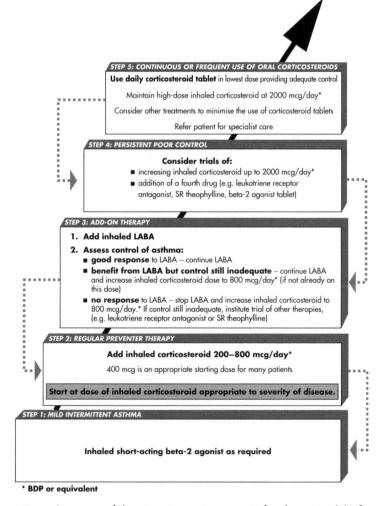

STEP 5: CONTINUOUS OR FREQUENT USE OF ORAL CORTICOSTEROIDS

Use daily corticosteroid tablet in lowest dose providing adequate control

Maintain high-dose inhaled corticosteroid at 2000 mcg/day*

Consider other treatments to minimise the use of corticosteroid tablets

Refer patient for specialist care

STEP 4: PERSISTENT POOR CONTROL

Consider trials of:
- increasing inhaled corticosteroid up to 2000 mcg/day*
- addition of a fourth drug (e.g. leukotriene receptor antagonist, SR theophylline, beta-2 agonist tablet)

STEP 3: ADD-ON THERAPY

1. **Add inhaled LABA**
2. **Assess control of asthma:**
   - **good response** to LABA – continue LABA
   - **benefit from LABA but control still inadequate** – continue LABA and increase inhaled corticosteroid dose to 800 mcg/day* (if not already on this dose)
   - **no response** to LABA – stop LABA and increase inhaled corticosteroid to 800 mcg/day.* If control still inadequate, institute trial of other therapies, (e.g. leukotriene receptor antagonist or SR theophylline)

STEP 2: REGULAR PREVENTER THERAPY

Add inhaled corticosteroid 200–800 mcg/day*

400 mcg is an appropriate starting dose for many patients

Start at dose of inhaled corticosteroid appropriate to severity of disease.

STEP 1: MILD INTERMITTENT ASTHMA

Inhaled short-acting beta-2 agonist as required

* **BDP or equivalent**

Figure 3.1 Summary of the stepwise management of asthma in adults from the British Thoracic Society/Scottish Intercollegiate Guidelines Network (BTS/SIGN) asthma management guideline.[1] (Reproduced with permission from the BMJ Publishing Group.) BDP, beclometasone diproprionate; LABA, long-acting beta-2 agonist; mcg, micrograms; SR, slow release.

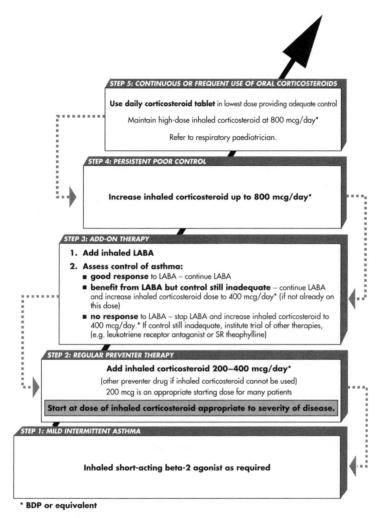

Figure 3.2   Summary of the stepwise management of asthma in children aged 5–12 years from the British Thoracic Society/Scottish Intercollegiate Guidelines Network (BTS/SIGN) asthma management guideline.[1] (Reproduced with permission from the BMJ Publishing Group.) BDP, beclometasone diproprionate; LABA, long-acting beta-2 agonist; mcg, micrograms; SR, slow release.

under 5 years of age). Treatment is started at a particular level according to the severity of the patient's symptoms. The aim is to achieve early control and maintain this by stepping up treatment as necessary and stepping down when control is good.

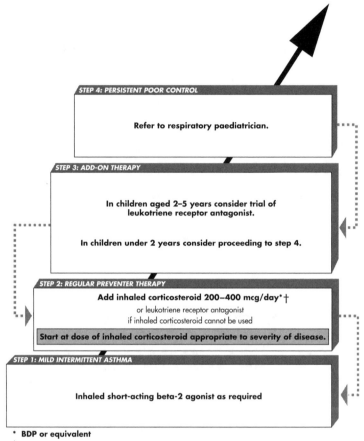

STEP 4: PERSISTENT POOR CONTROL

Refer to respiratory paediatrician.

STEP 3: ADD-ON THERAPY

**In children aged 2–5 years consider trial of
leukotriene receptor antagonist.**

In children under 2 years consider proceeding to step 4.

STEP 2: REGULAR PREVENTER THERAPY

Add inhaled corticosteroid 200–400 mcg/day* †

or leukotriene receptor antagonist
if inhaled corticosteroid cannot be used

Start at dose of inhaled corticosteroid appropriate to severity of disease.

STEP 1: MILD INTERMITTENT ASTHMA

Inhaled short-acting beta-2 agonist as required

* **BDP or equivalent**
† **Higher nominal doses may be required if drug delivery is difficult**

Figure 3.3 Summary of the stepwise management of asthma in children under 5 years of age, from the British Thoracic Society/Scottish Intercollegiate Guidelines Network (BTS/SIGN) asthma management guideline.[1] (Reproduced with permission from the BMJ Publishing Group.) BDP, beclometasone diproprionate; mcg, micrograms; SR, slow release.

Cultural and patient preferences should be taken into account in establishing a long-term treatment plan. Such a plan is often a compromise between the optimal prescribed medication and what the patient is prepared to take or can afford to take. Failure to consider these issues before prescribing treatments will result in poor concordance with the regimen and suboptimal or dreadful control (see Chapter 16).

Pharmacological therapy must be accompanied at every step by patient education and measures to control factors that contribute to the severity of the asthma. Ways to avoid trigger factors, the mode of action of medications and the use of inhalation devices should be explained to the patient clearly and repeatedly (see Chapter 8). All patients with asthma (and parents of children with asthma) should receive a written action plan that clearly indicates and differentiates the maintenance treatment and the quick reliever medication. This action plan should instruct the patient on what to do in the event of an exacerbation and support the verbal information provided.

If optimal control of asthma is not achieved and sustained at any step of the guideline (nocturnal symptoms, urgent visits to the doctor or an increased need for SABAs are key indications that asthma is not optimally controlled), several actions may be considered.[1]

- Patient concordance with the treatment regimen should be assessed.
- The patient's technique in using inhaled medications should be assessed to ensure that devices are being used correctly.
- A short course of oral prednisolone (40–50 mg daily for 5 days or until control is re-established) is often effective to regain control of asthma. If symptoms do not recur and pulmonary function remains normal, no additional therapy is necessary. However, if the 'prednisolone burst' does not control symptoms, is effective for only a short period of time (i.e. less than 1–2 weeks) or is repeated frequently, the patient should be managed according to the next step of the guideline.
- Other factors that diminish control may need to be identified and addressed. These factors include: the presence of a coexisting condition (e.g. sinusitis, rhinitis); a new or increased exposure to allergens; patient or family barriers to adequate self-management behaviours; psychosocial problems. In some cases, alternative diagnoses may need to be considered, such as vocal cord dysfunction.
- A step up to the next higher step of care may be necessary.

Continual monitoring of asthma control is essential to ensure that treatments are effective. Control can be monitored objectively by using a peak flow meter, by reviewing the need for SABAs or subjectively by assessing patient symptoms and activity levels. If control is not achieved with appropriate initial therapy, the treatment plan (and possible the diagnosis) should be re-evaluated.

Once control is achieved and sustained for a few months, a reduction in the pharmacological therapy is recommended to the lowest level that maintains control. As asthma is a variable disease, any changes in long-term treatments should be made after the patient has been observed for a sufficient length of time. An observation period of approximately 3 months seems to be appropriate to judge control of chronic asthma. External factors may change the control of asthma, for example high pollen counts, introduction of a new pet or starting smoking or passive smoking, which need to be considered when reviewing the patient's medication.

Step 1: Mild intermittent asthma

Mild intermittent asthma describes asthma in which the patient experiences episodes of symptoms (cough, wheezing or dyspnoea) less than once a week over a period of at least 3 months and the episodes are brief, generally lasting only a few hours to a few days. Between exacerbations the patient is symptom free and has a normal lung function. This category also includes patients with allergies who are occasionally exposed to the allergen that is responsible for causing their asthma, but who are completely symptom free and have normal lung function when not exposed to the allergen. This category also includes patients who have occasional exercise-induced asthma (EIA) (e.g. under bad weather circumstances).

SABAs, taken as needed to treat symptoms, are recommended as short-term reliever therapy for all patients with symptomatic asthma.[1] No long-term controller medications are required because the patient is asymptomatic and has normal lung function between episodes of asthma. Any exacerbations should be treated as such depending on their severity. If effective in relieving symptoms, intermittent use of a SABA can continue on an as-needed basis. If significant symptoms reccur or the SABA is required to relieve symptoms more than three times a week (with the exception of using a SABA for exacerbations caused by viral infections and for exercise-induced bronchospasm), treatment should be moved up to the next step of the guideline.[1] Patients with intermittent asthma who experience exercise-induced bronchospasm benefit from taking an inhaled SABA shortly before exercise. The BTS/SIGN guideline suggests that an inhaled anticholinergic, oral SABA or theophylline may be considered as alternatives to inhaled SABA, although these alternatives have a slower onset of action and/or a higher risk of side-effects.[1]

Inhaled SABAs should be prescribed for use on an as-needed rather than a regular basis. Randomised controlled trials have found that regular use of inhaled SABAs provides no additional clinical benefits compared with use 'as needed' and may worsen control of asthma.[3,4]

Two case-controlled studies found an association between increased asthma mortality and overuse of inhaled SABAs,[5,6] although the evidence does not establish causality, as overusing beta-2 agonists to treat frequent symptoms may simply indicate severe uncontrolled asthma in high-risk individuals. Inhaling a SABA on an as-needed basis is a useful indicator of disease control and allows the patient to judge how often they require rescue medication and how effective it is when administered. Patients with high usage of inhaled SABA should have their asthma management reviewed. Using two or more canisters of SABA per month or >10–12 puffs per day are markers of poorly controlled asthma.[1] Patients using high doses of beta-2 agonists are more likely to experience adverse effects, such as tremor, cramps, palpitations and headache. Beta-2 agonists can mask symptoms but do not change the underlying disease process. The administration of SABAs in the treatment of acute or chronic asthma is not a substitute for the early use of anti-inflammatory drugs. Some patients persist for too long using SABAs during an asthma exacerbation and do not seek medical help early enough. It is obvious that patients who rely on beta-2 agonists alone, which provides excellent symptomatic relief, may perceive their asthma to be improving, whereas in reality their delay in receiving anti-inflammatory medication may put them at risk. Once severe bronchoconstriction has occurred, inhaled SABAs can have little effect and anti-inflammatory drugs (i.e. corticosteroids) are needed. Failure to achieve a quick and sustained response to beta-2 agonist treatment during an exacerbation requires immediate medical attention.

Step 2: Introduction of regular preventer therapy

The BTS/SIGN guideline recommends that patients with persistent mild, moderate or severe asthma receive daily long-term preventer medication.[1] The most effective preventer medications are the ICSs as they diminish chronic airway inflammation and airway hyperresponsiveness.

ICSs target the inflamed airways directly, reducing oedema and the secretion of mucus into the airway. Many studies have now shown that early intervention with ICSs produces a far greater improvement in symptoms and lung function than increasing the dose of a SABA.

The exact threshold for introduction of ICS has never firmly been established. Recent studies have shown that patients with mild asthma (FEV_1 90% predicted) benefit from a low-dose ICS.[7,8] The BTS/SIGN guideline recommends the use of ICSs in patients with the following criteria:[9]

- an exacerbation of their asthma in the last 2 years
- using an inhaled SABA three times a week or more
- experiencing asthma symptoms three times a week or more, or waking one night a week.

Previous British asthma guidance suggested that the ICS should be started at a high dose to gain control quickly and then stepped down according to symptoms. However, in mild-to-moderate asthma this confers no benefit. The initiation dose should be appropriate to the severity of the disease and the dose titrated to the lowest dose at which effective control of asthma is maintained. This dose is usually 400 micrograms/day of beclometasone or equivalent in adults and 200 micrograms/day in children. Higher doses may be required initially in children under 5 years of age to compensate for ineffective drug delivery.

Many studies have compared the different ICSs although many are poorly designed; nevertheless, these studies suggest that the different ICS preparations are not equivalent on a per-puff or microgram basis. The effect of this in clinical practice is not known because there are few data directly comparing the preparations. Relative dosing for clinical comparability is affected by differences in topical potency, clinical effects at different doses, delivery device, bioavailability and patient factors, such as inspiratory flow rate. Taking into consideration these variables, dose equivalence has been suggested (See Management Focus, below). Budesonide and chlorofluorohydrocarbon (CFC)-containing

MANAGEMENT FOCUS

Dosages of inhaled corticosteroids equivalent to beclometasone, 200 micrograms/day		
	Ratio compared with beclometasone	Equivalent dosage (micrograms/day)
Budesonide (Pulmicort)	1:1	200
HFA-containing beclometasone (QVAR)[a]	1:2	100
Fluticasone (Flixotide)	1:2	100
Mometasone (Asmanex)	1:2	100

[a]chlorofluorohydrocarbon-free beclometasone inhaler.
HFA, hydrofluoroalkane-134a.

beclometasone are approximately equivalent in clinical practice (although there may be variations when different delivery devices are used) and a 1:1 ratio should be assumed when changing between these. If patients are switched from a budesonide or CFC-containing beclometasone inhaler to one containing hydrofluoroalkane-134a (HFA) as the propellant (CFC-free beclometasone), the total daily dose is halved. Fluticasone and the new ICS mometasone provide the same clinical effects as CFC-containing beclometasone and budesonide but at half the dosage. Once switched to a different ICS, the dose should be adjusted to meet the needs of the patient. However, to avoid systemic adverse effects, the minimum dose at which control of asthma is maintained should be used.

ICSs should be administered at least twice a day. Currently available ICSs are slightly more effective when taken twice rather than once daily[9] but there is little evidence of benefit for dosage frequencies of more than twice daily. Studies have shown that if good control is established, the same total daily dose of ICS can be given once a day rather than in divided doses, maintaining asthma control.

ICSs are the first-choice preventer drug. Alternatives are available but they should only be prescribed if an ICS is absolutely contra-indicated or if the patient refuses to take steroid preparations. Sustained-release theophylline is an alternative preventer medication. It is not preferred because it's modest clinical effectiveness as a preventer (theophylline is mainly a bronchodilator, see Chapter 13) must be balanced against concerns about potential toxicity and the need to measure plasma levels. Theophylline remains a therapeutic option for certain patients, especially when a tablet formulation is preferred. Leukotriene receptor antagonists, long-acting beta-2 agonists (LABAs) and sodium cromoglicate can also be considered as alternative long-term preventer medications. Leukotriene receptor antagonists have some clinical effects and have the advantage of being available in tablet form; however, they are not as effective as ICSs. LABAs have some beneficial effects but are not recommended for first-line preventer therapy and, in fact, should not be prescribed without an ICS.[10] Sodium cromoglicate is of some benefit in adults and is effective in children aged 5–12 years but there is no evidence to support its use in children under 5 years of age.[1]

Quick reliever medication must be available. Inhaled SABAs should be used as needed to relieve symptoms. Use of inhaled SABAs on a daily basis, or increasing use, indicates the need for additional therapy.

Step 3: Add-on therapy

Before a new drug is initiated, the prescriber should check the patient's concordance with medication and their inhaler technique. The presence of any trigger factors should be investigated and education provided on avoidance.

There is no precise dose of ICS at which the patient should be moved up to step 3, which involves adding additional treatments to the regimen. The addition of other treatment options to an ICS has been investigated at doses from 200 to 1000 micrograms/day of BDP or equivalent in adults and 400 micrograms/day in children. At step 3, increasing the dose of ICS above 800 micrograms beclometasone or equivalent is not recommended because this increases the risk of adverse effects and there is little increase in benefit. A trial of other treatments should be initiated before the dose of ICS is increased above 800 micrograms/day in adults or 400 micrograms/day in children.[1]

There are at least three options for initiating step 3 therapies (see Figure 3.4).

1.   Increase ICS to medium dose (≤800 micrograms/day of BDP or equivalent in adults or ≤400 micrograms/day in children).
2.   Add a long-acting bronchodilator to a low-to-medium dose of ICS.

Clinical evidence, from trials in over 3600 adult and adolescent patients, demonstrates the benefit of adding an inhaled LABA to an ICS compared with increasing the dose of ICS. A LABA should be tried in patients whose asthma is not well controlled on low doses of ICS, and the patient's outcome monitored. The clinical trials showed that LABAs improve outcomes such as lung function and symptoms and decrease exacerbations – outcomes that can be used to assess patients. If the treatment is successful, it should be continued. If there is partial response to the addition of a LABA, the dose of ICS should be increased to 800 micrograms/day of BDP or equivalent in adults (400 micrograms/day in children). If the treatment is unsuccessful, the LABA should be stopped and an alternative therapy tried. There is no difference in efficacy between giving the ICS and LABA in combination or in separate inhalers.[9]

3.   Add an alternative therapy (e.g. theophylline, leukotriene receptor antagonist or slow-release beta-2 agonist tablets).

The addition of short-acting anticholinergics is generally of no value and the addition of sodium cromoglicate is of marginal benefit.[1]

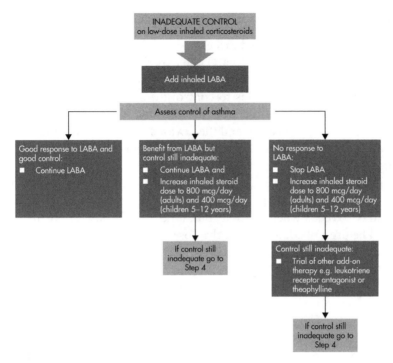

Figure 3.4   Summary of Step 3 of the British Thoracic Society/Scottish Collegiate Guidelines Network asthma management guideline: add-on therapy.[1] (Reproduced with permission from the BMJ Publishing Group.) LABA, long-acting beta-2 agonist; mcg, micrograms.

Step 4: Persistent poor control

For a small number of patients, control of asthma cannot be achieved by the combination of an SABA as needed, ICS (800 micrograms/daily of BDP or equivalent) and an additional drug, usually a LABA. There are few clinical trials to guide the prescriber to the best option at this step. The BTS/SIGN guideline recommends consideration of the following options:

- increase the dose of ICS to 2000 micrograms/day of BDP or equivalent (adults) or 800 micrograms/day (children aged 5–12 years)
- leukotriene receptor antagonist
- theophylline
- slow-release beta-2 agonist tablets

Step 5: Continuous or frequent use of oral steroids

Control of asthma as defined earlier may not be possible. Patients at step 5 have severe persistent asthma. They experience frequent severe exacerbations in spite of medication and their activities are limited. The aim of management at this step is to control the symptoms or gain the best possible control, achieve the best possible lung function, the least circadian (night to day) variation and the fewest side-effects from medication. In practice, treatment usually consists of a combination of various preventers (corticosteroids, leukotriene receptor antagonist) and reliever medications (SABA, LABA, methylxanthines). Patients usually require an oral corticosteroid (e.g. prednisolone) to maintain asthma control. This should be avoided when possible, but, if needed, the lowest possible dose should be prescribed. To reduce the dose or eliminate the steroid tablets, patients should be prescribed ICS (beclometasone or equivalent) up to 2000 microgram/day. Patients on long-term steroid tablets (e.g. longer than 3 months) or who require frequent courses of steroid tablets (e.g. three or four courses each year) will be at risk of systemic side-effects (see Chapter 12). These patients should be monitored carefully for the appearance of adverse effects (See Adverse Effects Focus, below).

Immunosuppressants – methotrexate, azathioprine,[11] ciclosporin and gold – can be given to reduce the requirements for steroid tablets in the long term but all have significant side-effects (see Management Focus, page 46). Although some of the compounds have corticosteroid-sparing effects, their use in asthma is complicated by highly variable effects, potential toxicity and limited clinical experience. Before considering immunosuppressants, it is important to re-evaluate a number of issues.

- The diagnosis needs to be confirmed and co-existing conditions, such as bronchiectasis, should be treated appropriately.

ADVERSE EFFECTS FOCUS

Monitoring of corticosteroid adverse effects
• Blood pressure
• Diabetes mellitus
• Osteoporosis
• Cataract screening in children
• Growth in children

- If asthma remains the diagnosis, the patient's current medication should be examined critically to ensure that it is appropriate according to the BTS/SIGN guideline in terms of drugs prescribed, route of administration and dosages. All should be optimised.
- Patient concordance with their regimen should be confirmed in any individual who remains symptomatic.

If, despite this approach, a patient's asthma remains poorly controlled then it is appropriate to consider systemic corticosteroids. These patients may benefit from a trial of immunosuppressants.

The complexity of a medication regimen for patients with severe asthma and the associated adverse effects are often factors in patient non-concordance, and this in turn complicates the control of asthma. Patients with severe persistent asthma may require particularly intensive patient education and guidance.

Stepping down

Stepping down of treatment once asthma is controlled is recommended. Reduction in therapy should be gradual because asthma can deteriorate at a highly variable rate and intensity. In general, the last medication added to the medical regimen should be the first medication to be reduced, but the severity of asthma, the side-effects of the treatment, the beneficial effect achieved and the patient's preferences should all be taken into account. Although guidelines for the rate of reduction and intervals for evaluation have not been established, the general opinion is that the dose of ICS should be reduced by 25–50% every 2–3 months to the lowest dose possible required to maintain control. A study in adults taking ICS at at least 900 micrograms per day of BDP or equivalent has shown that for patients whose asthma is stable, it is reasonable to try to halve the dose of inhaled steroids every 3 months.[12] Most patients with persistent asthma will require daily medication to suppress underlying airway inflammation. A patient's asthma may relapse when ICSs are discontinued completely. Regular review as treatment is reduced is essential.

Specific management problems

Occupational asthma

The aim of managing occupational asthma is to identify the cause and then to either remove the subject from exposure or remove the cause

Immunosuppressive/corticosteroid-sparing therapy
Note that these drugs are not licensed for the treatment of asthma

Drug	Mechanism of action	Suggested dosage[a]	Common side-effects	Notes
Methotrexate	Inhibits: • granulocyte chemotaxis • histamine release from basophils • actions of IL-1	15 mg once weekly	Nausea, abdominal discomfort, blood dyscrasias hepatic damage, pneumonitis	• Response is unpredictable • Perform full blood count, renal and liver function tests before starting treatment; repeat weekly until therapy is stabilised; thereafter every 2–3 months throughout treatment • In view of reports of blood dyscrasias and liver cirrhosis, patients should report all symptoms and signs suggestive of infection, especially sore throat
Ciclosporin A	Inhibits: • secretion of leukotrienes by mast cells and basophils • platelet activating factor • histamine • lymphocyte synthesis of cytokines • B cell synthesis of IgE • eosinophil activation	3–7.5 mg/kg daily	Nephrotoxicity, hypertension, hypertrichosis, increased susceptibility to infection, elevation of liver enzymes, gastrointestinal disturbances, hyperkalaemia, hypomagnesaemia, hypercholesterolaemia	• Results are often disappointing • Therapeutic plasma levels: 80–150 ng/ml • Because of the possibility of renal dysfunction or structural changes, serum creatinine should be measured at baseline and at 2-weekly intervals during the first 3 months of therapy and then at monthly intervals if creatinine remains stable • In view of the adverse effects, measure blood pressure, serum potassium and magnesium and blood lipids before treatment and thereafter as appropriate • The brand of ciclosporin to be dispensed should be specified by the prescriber, as preparations differ in bioavailabilty

Drug	Mechanism of action	Suggested dosage[a]	Common side-effects	Notes
Gold	Inhibits: • lymphocyte responses • prostaglandin synthesis • lysozymes • mast cell/basophil mediator relapse[b] • chemotaxis[b] • antibody synthesis[b] • release of IL-1 and IL-2[b]	Parenteral sodium aurothiomalate 25–50 mg once a week by intramuscular injection or oral auranofin 6 mg daily	Skin rashes, nephropathy, gastrointestinal disturbances (diarrhoea with or without nausea or abdominal pain). Reactions that resemble anaphylactoid effects have been reported and may occur after any course of therapy within the first 10 minutes of drug administration	• Side-effects limit use • Before starting treatment and again before each administration, urine should be tested for protein, skin inspected for rash and a full blood count performed • Gold therapy should be discontinued in the presence of blood disorders, gastrointestinal bleeding or unexplained protenuria • In view of the adverse effects, patients should be advised to tell the doctor immediately if sore throat, buccal ulceration, fever, infection, non-specific illness, unexplained bleeding or bruising, purpura, metallic taste or rashes develop
Normal Immunoglobulin	Variety of immunomodulatory roles	1–2 g/kg once a month	Headaches (mild and self-limiting), malaise, chills, fever, allergic reactions and rarely anaphylaxis	• Expensive • Indirect benefit in those with pre-existing immunoglobulin deficiency by preventing infection • Normal immunoglobulin may interfere with the immune response to live-virus vaccines, which should therefore only be given at least 3 weeks before or 3 months after an injection of normal immunoglobulin

continued overleaf

Management Focus (continued)

Drug	Mechanism of action	Suggested dosage[a]	Common side-effects	Notes
Anti-malarials (chloroquine and hydroxychloroquine)	Inhibition of phospholipase A_2	Hydroxychloroquine 400 mg/day Chloroquine (base) 15 mg/day (approximate equivalences: chloroquine base 150 mg = chloroquine sulphate 200 mg = chloroquine phosphate 250 mg)	Retinopathy, impairment of liver and renal function, gastrointestinal disturbances, rash, bone marrow suppression	• Renal and liver function should be assessed before treatment and the dose adjusted if either is impaired • Ophthalmological assessments should be done before use and at 3–6-month (chloroquine) or 12-month intervals (hydroxychloroquine) during use • Full blood counts should be performed regularly during extended treatment • Avoid in patients with epilepsy as convulsions have been reported in association with chloroquine • All patients on long-term hydroxychloroquine should undergo periodic examination of skeletal muscle function and tendon reflexes; the drug should be withdrawn if weakness occurs • There is no evidence to support the use of anti-malarials in asthma
Azathioprine	Incorporated into DNA and prevents cell division; mechanism by which this reduces immunosuppression is not fully understood	2 mg/kg daily	Bone marrow suppression, increased susceptibility to infection, hepatotoxicity, gastrointestinal disturbances	• Monitor full blood counts weekly during the first 8 weeks of therapy then every 1–3 months thereafter • Patients should report immediately any evidence of infection, unexpected bruising or bleeding or other manifestations of bone marrow depression • Monitor liver function • There is little evidence to support the use of azathioprine in asthma

Drug	Mechanism of action	Suggested dosage[a]	Common side-effects	Notes
Colchicine	• Inhibits neutrophils • Blocks release of IL-1 from lymphocytes • Intracellular levels of cAMP increased	0.5 mg twice daily	Diarrhoea common, neuropathy, myopathy	• There are few trials evaluating use of colchicine in asthma
Dapsone	Inhibits neutrophil burst and chemotaxis	100 mg twice daily	Haemolytic anaemia, methaemoglobulinaemia, agranulocytosis, gastrointestinal disturbances, hepatitis, neuropsychiatric reactions, skin rashe	• Monitor full blood count and renal function; perform liver function tests • Patients should know how to recognise signs of blood disorders and be advised to seek immediate medical attention if symptoms such as fever, sore throat, rash, mouth ulcers, purpura, bruising or bleeding develop • Evidence favouring the use of dapsone is outweighed by the potentially toxic side-effects

[a]based on current published literature.
[b]Auranofin only.
cAMP, cyclic adenosine monophosphate; IgE, immunoglobulin E; IL, interleukin.

from the workplace if possible. Wearing a facemask does not reduce symptoms of occupational asthma. Several studies have shown that the prognosis for workers with occupational asthma is worse for those who remain exposed for more than 1 year after symptoms develop, compared with those removed earlier. Removal from the causative agent should therefore occur within 12 months of the first work-related asthma symptom. Subjects who are unable to leave their job should minimise contact time with the causative agent and their asthma should be treated according to the BTS/SIGN guideline.[1]

Employers and their health and safety personnel should be aware of the large number of agents known to cause occupational asthma and the associated risk of exposure to such agents. The most frequently reported agents include isocyanates, flour and grain dust, colophony and fluxes, latex, animals, aldehydes and wood dust. Employers have legal responsibilities to control the causative agents of occupational asthma. In the UK these requirements come under the auspices of The Control of Substances Hazardous to Health Regulations (COSHH) regulated by the Health and Safety Executive. In summary, employers must:

- assess the risks and decide what precautions are needed
- prevent or adequately control exposure by elimination or substitution if this is not possible by engineering controls such as enclosure and extraction, or by using respiratory protective equipment
- ensure control measures are used and maintained
- monitor exposure regularly
- provide health surveillance to at-risk groups.

If workers suspect they have occupational asthma, they should be advised to speak to their general practitioner. Compensation is available from the Department of Social Security for most occupational lung diseases (known as 'Prescribed Diseases').

Exercise-induced asthma

The usual approach to the management of EIA is prevention. For most patients who have normal lung function, EIA will be prevented by taking a SABA 10–15 minutes before exercise. These usually provide 60–70% protection against EIA when exercise is performed within 30 minutes of taking the drug.[13,14]

The LABAs salmeterol and formoterol also provide good protection against EIA. For those with mild EIA, these LABAs may afford protection for 8–12 hours, although patients with moderate-to-severe EIA may be protected for only 4–6 hours.[14,15] However, tolerance to their protection effect against exercise has been shown to develop when taken on a twice-daily basis for 1 month.[16–18]

Oral bronchodilators such as theophyllines, leukotriene receptor antagonists and beta-2 agonist tablets have been shown to give protection against EIA.[1] Leukotriene receptor antagonists provide prolonged protection against EIA and the development of tolerance has not been demonstrated.[1] EIA may be prevented by inhaling sodium cromoglicate; it has an immediate onset of action and duration of action of 1.5–2.5 hours. There are no reports of tolerance developing to the protective effects and it can be inhaled many times a day.

In many patients, EIA is a symptom of poorly controlled asthma. Treatment with an ICS usually gains control of their asthma and reduces the severity of EIA within days or weeks.[19,20] If patients are already taking an ICS, the dose may need to be titrated to inhibit EIA. Anticholinergics, ketotifen and antihistamines do not given protection against EIA at normal doses.

Aspirin-sensitive asthma

In general, aspirin-sensitive asthma is managed in the same way as other types of asthma. Some patients may benefit from the addition of an leukotriene receptor antagonist but the response is variable and needs to be judged on an individual basis.

Desensitisation to aspirin is possible by graded introduction of aspirin and staying on a daily maintenance dose. In some patients, desensitisation improves nasal symptoms and asthma control and reduces the recurrence of nasal polyps.[21] Desensitisation is also indicated if the patient requires aspirin or a non-steroidal anti-inflammatory for cardiovascular prophylaxis or the treatment of arthritis. This should only be done under the supervision of a specialist with experience of the procedure.

Allergic bronchopulmonary aspergillosis

Aspergillus fumigatus appears in many places in the environment, which makes the fungus difficult to avoid. The mainstay of treatment for allergic bronchopulmonary aspergillosis (ABPA) remains oral corticosteroids,[1] though this does not prevent exacerbations completely and may not prevent the decline in lung function. Prednisolone taken initially in high doses and then over a long period of time at lower doses may provide symptomatic benefit. The oral route is recommended. The azole antifungal drugs may be helpful in controlling ABPA.[22] They are active against *A. fumigatus* and modify the immunological activation associated with ABPA. Short-term studies suggest that these drugs may improve clinical outcomes when added to standard therapy, at least over a period of 16 weeks.[22] The BTS/SIGN guideline recommends a 4 month trial of itraconazole in adults with ABPA.[9]

Corticosteroid-resistant asthma

True corticosteroid-resistant asthma is a challenge to manage. It is essential that the diagnosis of asthma is confirmed before treatment is initiated. Patients with corticosteroid-resistant asthma show a disappointing response even to large and prolonged doses of oral or intravenous corticosteroids. Higher doses may be required but it is important to note that these patients are at risk of developing adverse effects from treatment. Patients with corticosteroid-resistant asthma should be treated according to the BTS/SIGN guideline for the management of asthma. Specific pharmacotherapy, as in asthma that is responsive to corticosteroids, is incremental depending upon severity. Bronchodilatation is the mainstay of therapy; however, immunosuppression and the use of the leukotriene receptor antagonists may be effective in certain patients. It is essential to detect and improve any poor concordance with medications and to optimise a delivery system for inhaled medication that the patient finds effective, acceptable and easy to use.

Vaccinations

Pneumococcal vaccination

Pneumococcus is the common name for the gram-positive bacterium *Streptococcus pneumoniae*, which is a major cause of a variety of common and serious infections. It is estimated to affect 1 in 1000 adults every year, with 10–20% mortality.[23] The risk of infection is greatest in immunocompromised individuals and in immunocompetent patients with chronic conditions such as cardiovascular disease, chronic pulmonary disease or diabetes. The UK Department of Health recommends that patients with chronic lung disease – including asthma – are vaccinated against pneumococcal infection. However, few high-quality studies have assessed the effects of pneumococcal vaccination in reducing morbidity and mortality from pneumococcal disease in people with asthma. A Cochrane review identified only one randomised controlled trial designed to test the efficacy of prophylactic sulfisoxazole and pneumococcal vaccination in reducing the incidence of otitis media in children with asthma.[24] This trial showed some benefit in reducing asthma exacerbations in children who had recurrent otitis media, but the trial methodology was deemed poor. The review concluded that the role of pneumococcal vaccination for people with asthma is unclear, and there is not enough evidence to warrant the recommendation of routine vaccination for all people with asthma.

Influenza vaccination

Influenza is one of the few respiratory illnesses for which vaccination is available. Respiratory infections of viral and bacterial origin are believed to be important causes of exacerbations in children with asthma. However, influenza infection accounts for only a small percentage of asthma exacerbations; in a study involving children aged 9–11 years old with asthma, influenza infection was identified in only a small number of exacerbations whereas the common cold virus was implicated in 80% of reported exacerbations.[25]

A systematic review of the efficacy of influenza vaccination in healthy adults concluded that the recommended inactivated parenteral influenza vaccines are effective in reducing serologically confirmed cases of influenza A in 68% of cases; however, the efficacy in reducing cases of clinical influenza was only 24%.[26]

Adverse reactions to influenza vaccination are usually mild and are restricted to myalgia and local redness and tenderness although there has been debate as to whether vaccination induces exacerbations in patients with asthma. A systematic review has examined whether influenza vaccination increased the risk of asthma exacerbations.[27] The review, which assessed findings from two large crossover studies using split virus or surface antigen influenza vaccination, found that that the likelihood of an asthma exacerbation immediately following influenza vaccination was very low.[28,29] The systematic review also examined whether influenza vaccination was effective in preventing asthma exacerbations. Data from randomised controlled trials assessing the protective effect of influenza vaccination in asthma are limited but, on the basis of available data, the review found that vaccination was not associated with a reduction in asthma exacerbations from influenza infection.

However, people with asthma are at increased risk of severe illness or death from influenza. All studies show that a large proportion of the increased morbidity and mortality in influenza epidemics is in those with long-term respiratory disease, which includes asthma. The benefits of vaccination are likely to outweigh the risks. The Joint Committee on Vaccination suggests that priority should be given to those requiring continuous or repeated use of inhaled or systemic corticosteroids or with previous exacerbations requiring hospital admission.

References

1. British Thoracic Society/Scottish Intercollegiate Guidelines Network. British Guideline on the Management of Asthma. *Thorax* 2003; 58 (Suppl I): S1–S94.
2. A general practitioner (medical editor of the home doctor and the household encyclopaedia). *The Illustrated Family Doctor*. London, 1934.
3. Sears MR, Taylor DR, Print CG, *et al*. Regular inhaled beta-agonist treatment in bronchial asthma. *Lancet* 1990; 336: 1391–1396.
4. Dennis SM, Sharp SJ, Vickers MR, *et al*. Regular inhaled salbutamol and asthma control: the TRUST randomised trial. *Lancet* 2000; 355: 1675–1679.
5. Spitzer WO, Suissa S, Ernst P, *et al*. The use of beta-2-agonists and the risk of death and near death from asthma. *N Engl J Med* 1992; 326: 501–506.
6. Crane J, Pearce N, Flatt A, *et al*. Prescribed fenoterol and death from asthma in New Zealand 1981–1983: case control study. *Lancet* 1989; 1: 917–922.
7. O'Byrne PM, Barnes PJ, Rodriguez-Roisin R, *et al*. Low dose inhaled budesonide and formoterol in mild persistent asthma: the OPTIMA randomised trial. *Am J Respir Crit Care Med* 2001; 164: 1392–1397.
8. Pauwels RA, Pederson S, Busse WW, *et al*. Early intervention with budesonide in mild persistent asthma: a randomised, double blind trial. *Lancet* 2003; 361 (9363): 1071–1076.
9. British Thoracic Society/Scottish Intercollegiate Guidelines Network. British Guideline on the Management of Asthma. Revised November 2005 (www.brit-thoracic.org.uk).
10. Salmeterol (Serevent) and formoterol (Oxis) in asthma management. *Curr Probl Pharmacovigilance* 2003; 29: 5.
11. Dean T, Dewey A, Bara A, *et al*. Azathioprine as an oral corticosteroid sparing agent for asthma. *The Cochrane Library*, issue 4. Chichester: John Wiley & Sons, 2003 (www.thecochranelibrary.com).
12. Hawkins G, McMahon AD, Twaddle S, *et al*. Stepping down inhaled corticosteroids in asthma: randomised controlled trial. *BMJ* 2003; 326(7399): 1115.
13. Anderson SD, Moreton AR, Lambert S, *et al*. Comparison of the bronchoprotective effect of single doses of Albuterol administered by Diskus dry powder inhaler and by metered dose inhaler against exercise-induced bronchoconstriction. *Am J Respir Crit Care Med* 1999; 153: A879.
14. Anderson SD, Rodwell LT, Du Toit J, *et al*. Duration of protection of inhaled salmeterol in exercise-induced asthma. *Chest* 1991; 100: 1254–1260.
15. Kemp JP, Dockhorn RJ, Busse WW, *et al*. Prolonged effect of inhaled

salmeterol against exercise-induced bronchospasm. *Am J Respir Crit Care Med* 1994; 150: 1612–1615.

16. Ramage L, Lipworth BJ, Ingram CG, *et al.* Reduced protection against exercise induced bronchoconstriction after chronic dosing with salmeterol. *Respir Med* 1994; 88: 363–368.

17. Simons FE, Gerstner TV, Cheang MS. Tolerance to the bronchoprotective effect of salmeterol in adolescents with exercise-induced asthma using concurrent inhaled glucocorticoid treatment. *Pediatrics* 1997; 99: 655–659.

18. Nelson JA, Strauss L, Skowronshi M, *et al.* Effect of long-term salmeterol treatment on exercise-induced asthma. *N Engl J Med* 1998; 339: 141–146.

19. Adams NP, Bestall JB, Jones PW. Inhaled beclometasone versus placebo for chronic asthma (Cochrane Review). *The Cochrane Library*, issue 3. Chichester: John Wiley & Sons, 2001 (www.thecochranelibrary.com).

20. Adams N, Bestall J, Jones PW. Inhaled fluticasone proprionate for chronic asthma (Cochrane Review). *The Cochrane Library*, issue 3. Chichester: John Wiley & Sons, 2001 (www.thecochranelibrary.com).

21. Stevenson DD, Hankammer MA, Mathison DA, *et al.* Aspirin desensitization treatment of aspirin-sensitive patients with rhinosinusitis-asthma: long-term outcomes. *J Allergy Clin Immunol* 1996; 98: 751–758.

22. Wark PAB, Gibson PG, Wilson AJ. Azoles for allergic bronchopulmonary aspergillosis associated with asthma. *The Cochrane Library*, issue 3. Chichester: John Wiley & Sons, 2004 (www.thecochranelibrary.com).

23. Chiodini J. Immunisation against pneumococcal disease can save lives. *Guidelines in Practice* 2002; 5(9): 48–53.

24. Sheikh A, Alves B, Dhami S. Pneumococcal vaccine for asthma. *The Cochrane Library*, issue 1. Chichester: John Wiley & Sons, 2002 (www.thecochrane library.com).

25. Johnston SL, Pattemore PK, Sanderson G, *et al.* Community study of role of viral infections in exacerbations of asthma in 9–11 year old children. *BMJ* 1995; 310: 1225–1229.

26. Demicheli V, Jefferson T, Rivetti D, *et al.* Prevention and early treatment of influenza in healthy adults. *Vaccine* 2000; 18: 957–1030.

27. Cates CJ, Jefferson TO, Bara AI, Rowe BH. Vaccines for preventing influenza in people with asthma. *The Cochrane Library*, issue 4. Chichester: John Wiley & Sons, 2003 (www.thecochranelibrary.com).

28. Nicholson KG, Nguyen-Van-Tam JS, Ahmed AH, *et al.* Randomised placebo-controlled crossover trial on effect of inactivated influenza vaccine on pulmonary function in asthma. *Lancet* 1998; 351: 326–331.

29. American Lung Association and Asthma Clinical Research Centers. The safety of inactivated influenza vaccine in adults and children with asthma. *N Engl J Med* 2001; 345: 1529–1536.

4

Management of acute asthma

Acute severe asthma is a major economic and health burden. In 2002, there were over 1400 deaths from asthma in the UK.[1] It is estimated that, on average, one person dies from asthma every 7 hours. However, approximately 75% of admissions to hospital are avoidable and as many as 90% of the deaths from asthma are preventable.[2] In many countries, asthma mortality increased from the 1960s to the second half of the 1980s, reached a plateau and has subsequently declined.[3] This recent downwards trend may reflect increased awareness of the signs and symptoms of acute asthma by patients and healthcare professionals and better management in primary care.

All patients with asthma are at risk of exacerbations, described by terms like 'acute asthma', 'asthma attack' and 'status asthmaticus'. The severity of exacerbations ranges from mild to life threatening. Deterioration usually progresses over hours, days or weeks; however, a few patients have sudden (over minutes) unexpected increases in airway obstruction. Approximately 90% of asthma exacerbations severe enough to warrant hospital admission develop over a period of 6 hours or more.[2] In one study, over 80% developed over more than 48 hours.[2] This observation suggests that in many patients there is a window of opportunity for recognition and reversal of this period of deterioration. Although sudden death is infrequent, it is useful practice to assume that every exacerbation is potentially fatal. Morbidity and mortality are most often associated with failure to appreciate the severity of an exacerbation, resulting in inadequate emergency treatment and delay in referring to hospital. Many patients coming to hospital with an acute severe exacerbation of asthma have received little or no treatment and others have only been given extra doses of beta-2 agonists in addition to their usual medication. Most studies of the factors relating to death from asthma have found inadequate treatment to be an important factor and in most patients who die from asthma there is a background of chronic under-treatment for various reasons; inadequate management of the final episode is due about equally to delay on the part of the patient in seeking help and inadequate treatment from the physician.

Deaths from asthma have been attributed to inappropriate prescribing of medications such as beta-blockers, non-steroidal anti-inflammatory drugs (NSAIDs), sedatives and even beta-2 agonists. Non-selective beta-blockers can cause bronchospasm and exacerbate asthma in susceptible individuals. Even non-selective beta-blocker ophthalmic solutions can be absorbed systemically and cause bronchospasm. If a patient with asthma requires a beta-blocker, a cardioselective beta-blocker should be chosen (e.g. atenolol, bisoprolol, metoprolol, nebivolol). These beta-blockers have less effect on bronchial beta-2 adrenoceptors and are therefore relatively *cardioselective*; they are, however, not *cardiospecific*. Adults with asthma should be questioned about episodes of bronchospasm associated with ingestion of aspirin or other NSAIDs. If a reaction has occurred, the patient should be warned about the dangers of a fatal exacerbation with use of these drugs. Patients with severe asthma or nasal polyps should also receive counselling about the potential of NSAIDs to cause a fatal exacerbation.[6,7] Evidence in the medical literature suggests that patients with asthma who take antipsychotics or sedatives are at increased risk of serious complications of their asthma. A number of mechanisms are potentially responsible for this association. Non-causal factors include patient characteristics (e.g. indication for antipsychotic use, non-concordance with asthma therapy, risk-taking behaviour and family dysfunction) and treatment issues (including differential prescribing and the quality of medical care). The main causal mechanism involves depression of the central nervous system and impaired respiratory drive resulting from sedation during an acute asthma attack. Certainly, the use of sedatives in non-intubated patients with asthma is associated with increased mortality and the need for mechanical ventilation.

It has been suggested that cardiac arrhythmias may contribute to some of the observed mortality from asthma. The risk is theoretically increased by hypokalaemia and the prolongation of the QT interval secondary to the administration of beta-2 agonists in high doses.[6] However, this could be explained by the fact that more severe asthma requires more treatment and is associated with a higher death rate despite treatment, not because of it. Most deaths are not drug induced but are related to the pathology of the disease: patients with fatal asthma almost invariably have extensive airflow limitation and hypoxaemia.

The Risk Factors Focus on page 59 highlights the behavioural and psychosocial factors that have been linked to deaths or near-deaths in

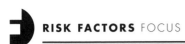

Risk factors for near-fatal or fatal asthma[2-5]

- Previous near-fatal asthma (e.g. previous ventilation or respiratory acidosis)
- Previous hospital admission for asthma
- Repeated attendances at emergency department for asthma care
- Failure to attend appointments
- Self-discharge from hospital
- Requirement for three or more classes of asthma medication
- Excessive use of inhalers with decreasing response
- Heavy use of beta-2 agonists
- Poor concordance with treatments or monitoring
- Lack of asthma action (self-management) plan
- Refractory (brittle) asthma
- Anxiety and depression, other psychiatric illness or deliberate self-harm
- Obesity
- Learning difficulties
- Social isolation
- Illicit drug use or alcohol abuse
- Disease denial
- Severe domestic, marital or legal stress
- Unemployment
- Shortness of breath that may have developed over hours or days
- Upper respiratory tract infection or exposure to an irritant atmosphere
- Personal or passive smoking

---

patients with asthma.[2-5] All health professionals must be aware that patients with severe asthma and one or more adverse psychosocial factors are at risk of death.

Mortality and morbidity from asthma exacerbations can be reduced by educating the patient about their condition and treatments, encouraging self-management (see Chapter 8) and improving the organisation of patient care in both primary and secondary care[2] (see Management Focus, page 60).

Pathology of acute asthma

The pathology of the airways in patients who have died during a severe asthma exacerbation has been described extensively. The pathology suggests two main types of acute asthma exacerbations. The most frequent, at least in asthma deaths, is caused by severe inflammation.

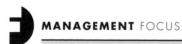

MANAGEMENT FOCUS

Recommended interventions to reduce asthma morbidity and mortality

---

Many patients with asthma and all patients with severe asthma

- Correct interpretation of warning symptoms at home
- Understanding of an agreed action plan
- Correct treatment at home
- Recognition when medical review or hospital treatment is needed

Primary care physician

- Correct evaluation
- Correct treatment
- Recognition of when referral to hospital is required (any patient with features of acute severe or life-threatening asthma; other factors, such as failure to respond to treatment, social circumstances or concomitant disease may warrant hospital referral)
- Register of patients at high risk of a fatal or a near-fatal attack
- Follow-up of high-risk patients if they do not attend for appointments at asthma clinic
- Avoid prescribing beta-blockers (including eye drops) and non-steroidal anti-inflammatory drugs for patients with asthma

Hospital

- Correct evaluation
- Correct criteria for admission to hospital[3]
  - Any patient with any feature of a life-threatening or near-fatal attack
  - Any patient with any feature of a severe attack persisting after initial treatment
  - Any patient whose PEF is greater than 75% best or predicted 1 hour after initial treatment but who still has significant symptoms, are non-concordant with medicines, live alone, have psychological problems, physical disability or learning difficulties, previous near-fatal or refractory asthma, present at night or are pregnant should be considered for admission to hospital.
- Patients should be managed in specialist rather than general units. Patients attending hospital with an acute exacerbation of asthma should be reviewed by clinicians with particular expertise in asthma management, preferably within 30 days.
- Correct treatment
- Recognition when transfer to intensive therapy unit is required
- Correct timing of discharge from hospital
- Correct follow-up and modification of treatment: a respiratory specialist should follow up patients admitted with severe asthma for at least 1 year after the admission; patients who have had near-fatal asthma or brittle asthma should remain under specialist supervision indefinitely

Airflow obstruction in these patients is due as much to mucus plugging as to airway smooth muscle spasm. The lungs of such patients are grossly overinflated, mainly because of the presence of plugs obstructing the small and medium airways. These plugs are composed of inflammatory cells, such as eosinophils and neutrophils, together with mucus and exuded plasma. Basophils are also found in increased numbers in fatal disease. The airway smooth muscle is hypertrophied and in a contracted state. The airway wall is grossly thickened, with vasodilated bronchial vessels, oedema and a gross infiltration of inflammatory cells, consisting of eosinophils, neutrophils and lymphocytes. The area of the airway wall in fatal cases has been reported to be increased by 10–100% over that seen in non-fatal disease and by 50–300% over that seen in non-asthmatic control subjects.[8,9] Thus, patients who have died with acute severe asthma have usually died of asphyxia. The pathology of acute asthma is illustrated in Figure 4.1.

The second main type of acute asthma exacerbation occurs in more patients prone to anaphylaxis. There is relatively little inflammation and most of the obstruction appears to result from airway smooth muscle spasm.

Causes of exacerbations

The cause of an exacerbation of asthma cannot be determined with any degree of certainty in many cases but exacerbations result from a number of factors (see Risk Factors Focus, page 63).

In many cases there is evidence of an upper respiratory tract infection, usually viral, before the exacerbation. Viruses induce an inflammatory response in the airways of patients with asthma. Exposure to allergens can also cause exacerbations in allergic asthmatics. Offending allergens, such as pollens or fungal spores occurring alone or in combination, have been linked to clusters of asthma exacerbations occurring at the time of thunderstorms in the UK.[10–14] Increased asthma morbidity during thunderstorms has been reported sporadically over the past two decades. On July 6th and 7th, 1983, the number of patients with asthma presenting to the emergency departments of eight Birmingham hospitals averaged 50 over the 2-day period, compared with a usual average of 10.[12] The increase in patient visits was associated with an increase in airborne fungal spores, particularly *Sporobolomyces* and *Didymella* species, and a decrease in pollen. Airborne pollutants represented by smoke and sulphur dioxide were not believed to be unusually elevated. The authors of the report

Cross section of normal lung

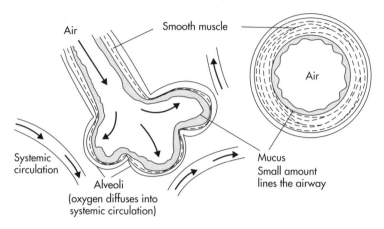

Cross section of the lung during an asthma exacerbation

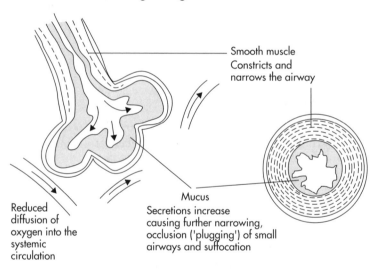

Figure 4.1 Cross-section of a normal healthy lung (top) and the pathological changes that occur in the lung during an acute asthma exacerbation (bottom).

suggested that asthma may have been caused by an increased release of fungal spores during the initial rainfall. During a thunderstorm 11 years later (June 24th and 25, 1994), the number of patients presenting with asthma or other airways diseases to emergency departments in the London area increased 10-fold. 'Out-of-hours' calls to primary care also increased during this time in south and east England.[13] This thunderstorm was described as unusually large and

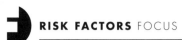

RISK FACTORS FOCUS

Causes of acute exacerbations of asthma

- Inhaled allergens
  - Patients often have a history of atopy
  - The severity of asthma has been correlated with the number of positive skin-prick test results
- Viral infection
- Air pollutants (e.g. dust, cigarette smoke, industrial pollutants)
- Medications, such as beta-blockers, aspirin and non-steroidal anti-inflammatory drugs
- Gastro-oesophageal reflux disease
  - Studies indicate that reflux of gastric contents with or without aspiration can trigger asthma in susceptible children and adults
  - Animal studies have shown that the instillation of even minute amounts of acid into the distal oesophagus can result in marked increases in intrathoracic pressure and airway resistance. This response is thought to be due to vagal and sympathetic neural responses.
- Cold temperature
- Exercise

multicentred, and was associated with reduced temperatures and severe wind gusting.[14,15]

Clinical presentation

Asthmatic patients often have isolated symptoms of asthma that are transient and subside quickly or are easily treated with one or two puffs of their short-acting beta-2 agonist inhaler. However, some patients have recurrent symptoms of asthma that are only partially treated by their reliever medication. Such episodes of poor control are often the prelude to an acute exacerbation of asthma. Acute severe asthma may progress over a period of days, hours or even minutes and can be life-threatening.

Clinically, an exacerbation is characterised by shortness of breath of varying degrees of severity, tachypnoea, chest tightness, wheezing, coughing and inability to speak in full sentences, although no sign or symptom is uniformly present. Dyspnoea is absent in 17–18% of cases[16] and wheezing is absent in 5%.[16] The absence of signs and symptoms does not exclude a severe attack, and wheezing is a poor indicator of functional impairment – it often increases as the obstruction resolves, allowing the flow of air through the airway. A more important indication of the severity of the asthma exacerbation is the absence of wheezing and/or the nature of the sounds. A silent chest represents a serious attack (see Diagnostic Focus, page 65).

In addition, the distribution of ventilation and perfusion and altered blood gases is abnormal in patients with severe asthma exacerbations. Patients with marked obstruction and significant lung hyperinflation can have electrocardiographic evidence of pulmonary hypertension, right ventricular pressure, reduced cardiac output, hypotension and poor peripheral perfusion. Typical blood gas abnormalities seen in acute asthma consist of a combination of hypoxaemia, hypocapnia and respiratory alkalosis. Measurement of oxygen saturation (SpO_2) with a pulse oximeter is necessary in acute severe asthma to determine the adequacy of oxygen therapy and the need for arterial blood gas (ABG) measurement (patients with SpO_2 <92%, or other features of life-threatening asthma require ABG measurement). Generally, the more severe the obstruction, the lower the SpO_2 and arterial oxygen tension (PaO_2). During an acute attack, patients generally hyperventilate, causing a reduction in the arterial carbon dioxide tension ($PaCO_2$). As the patient becomes tired and their breathing slows, the $PaCO_2$ starts to normalise, which should be viewed as a sign of impending respiratory failure and treated as such. The majority of patients have respiratory alkalosis although metabolic acidosis may be seen with extreme airflow limitation.

Differential diagnosis

A number of conditions may mimic or complicate the diagnosis of acute asthma. The absence of a history of asthma, particularly in an adult, should be treated with care and an alternative diagnosis considered.

- Congestive heart failure may present with acute shortness of breath accompanied by wheezing.
- The most common and difficult diagnosis is the differentiation of asthma from chronic obstructive pulmonary disease (see Diagnostic Focus p. 28 Chapter 2).
- Laryngeal, tracheal or bronchial obstruction may produce shortness of breath and localised wheezing that often mimics asthma.
- Recurrent small pulmonary emboli may manifest as attacks of shortness of breath and, very rarely, wheezing heard on careful auscultation.
- Recurrent attacks of shortness of breath at rest may be due to the hyperventilation syndrome.

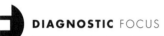

DIAGNOSTIC FOCUS

Severity of acute asthma exacerbations and associated signs and symptoms in adults and children

Nature of asthma	Adults and children over 12 years of age	Children 2–12 years of age
Moderate	Increasing symptoms PEF >50–70% best or predicted No features of acute severe asthma	Increasing symptoms PEF >50–70% best or predicted (attempt to measure PEF in all children over 6 years of age) No features of acute severe asthma
Acute severe	Any one of: • PEF 33–50% • Respiratory rate ≥25 breaths/minute • Heart rate ≥110 beats/minute • Inability to complete sentences in one breath	Any one of: • PEF 33–50% • Respiratory rate: children >5 years of age – >30 breaths/minute; 2–5 years of age – >50 breaths/minute • Heart rate: children >5 years of age – >120 beats/minute; 2–5 years of age >130 beats/minute • Inability to complete sentences in one breath or too breathless to talk or feed
Life-threatening	Any one of the following in a patient with severe asthma: • PEF <33% best or predicted • SpO_2 <92% • PaO_2 <8 kPa • Normal $PaCO_2$ (4.6–6.0 kPa) • Silent chest • Cyanosis • Poor respiratory effort • Bradycardia • Dysrhythmia • Hypotension • Exhaustion • Confusion • Coma	Any one of the following in a patient with severe asthma: • Silent chest • Cyanosis • Poor respiratory effort • Hypotension • Exhaustion • Confusion • Coma

continued overleaf

Diagnostic Focus *continued*		
Nature of asthma	Adults and children over 12 years of age	Children 2–12 years of age
Near-fatal	Raised $PaCO_2$ and/or requiring mechanical ventilation with raised inflation pressures	Fall in heart rate in life-threatening asthma
Refractory (brittle)	**Type 1** Wide PEF variability (>40% diurnal variation for >50% of the time over a period of >150 days) despite intense therapy	
	Type 2 Sudden severe attacks on a background of apparently well controlled asthma	

$PaCO_2$, arterial carbon dioxide tension; PaO_2, arterial oxygen tension; PEF, peak expiratory flow; SpO_2, oxygen saturation.

Treatment of acute asthma in adults

The hospital management of acute asthma in adults according to the British Thoracic Society/Scottish Intercollegiate Guidelines Network (BTS/SIGN) asthma management guideline is illustrated in Figure 4.2.

Aims of treatment

The severity of an asthma exacerbation determines the treatment. The goals of treatment can be summarised as: maintenance of adequate arterial oxygen saturation with supplemental oxygen, relief of airflow obstruction with repetitive administration of rapid-acting inhaled bronchodilators (beta-2 agonists and anticholinergics), reduction of airway inflammation and prevention of future relapses with early administration of systemic corticosteroids.

Oxygen

Hypoxaemia is the most common cause of death in asthma exacerbations. High concentrations of oxygen (usually 40–60%) should be given to correct hypoxaemia. There is little risk of inducing hypercapnia with high-flow oxygen in acute asthma, unlike in patients with chronic obstructive pulmonary disease. Even the nebuliser should be driven using oxygen if possible. Hypercapnia indicates the development of near-fatal asthma and the need for emergency intervention. The goal of treatment should be to maintain SpO_2 at 92% or higher.

Beta-2 agonist bronchodilators

Beta-2 agonists should be given in high doses and as early as possible to relieve bronchospasm. There is no evidence for any differences in efficacy between salbutamol and terbutaline.[3] Table 4.1 summarises the prescribing information for adults, children and infants with acute asthma exacerbations.

With regard to use of beta-2 agonists, there are four areas of debate.

1. *Metered-dose inhaler (MDI) with spacer versus nebulised administration.* An MDI and large-volume spacer provide an effective alternative to a nebuliser in mild-to-moderate acute asthma. In acute asthma with life-threatening features, the nebulised route driven by oxygen is the preferred method of administration.

2. *Parenteral versus inhaled therapy.* The inhaled route provides a faster onset of action, fewer adverse effects and is more effective than parenteral routes of administration in the majority of cases (subcutaneous route excluded from meta-analysis).[17] Parenteral beta-2 agonists in addition to inhaled beta-2 agonists may have a role in ventilated patients and patients in extremis in whom nebulised therapy may fail (e.g. patient is coughing excessively), but the evidence base for this is limited.

3. *Doses and intervals of administration.* The BTS/SIGN asthma management guideline recommends the use of high and repeated doses (e.g. salbutamol, 5 mg, in adults), inducing maximal stimulation of beta-2 adrenoceptors with minimal side-effects. However, there is a body of evidence to suggest that administering low doses of beta-2 agonist after the initial high dose is as effective. A study in adults comparing nebulised salbutamol, 5 mg administered every 4 hours, versus salbutamol, 2.5–5 mg, on demand, found that on-demand dosing was associated with reductions in the amount of drug delivered, incidence of adverse effects and possibly length of hospital stay (hospital stay 3.7 days with on-demand dosing versus 4.7 days with regular salbutamol).[18] Another study concluded that there is no advantage to the routine administration of doses of salbutamol higher than 2.5 mg every 20 minutes.[19] This study did not enrol sufficient numbers of patients with severe asthma, so it is

Management of acute severe asthma in adults in hospital

Features of acute severe asthma

- Peak expiratory flow (PEF) 33-50% of best (use % predicted if recent best unknown)
- Can't complete sentences in one breath
- Respirations ≥ 25 breaths/min
- Pulse ≥ 110 beats/min

Life threatening features

- PEF < 33% of best or predicted
- SpO_2 < 92%
- Silent chest, cyanosis, or feeble respiratory effort
- Bradycardia, dysrhythmia, or hypotension
- Exhaustion, confusion, or coma

If a patient has any life threatening features, measure arterial blood gases. No other investigations are needed for immediate management.

Blood gas markers of a life threatening attack:
- Normal (4.6-6 kpa, 35-45 mmHg) $PaCO_2$
- Severe hypoxia: Pao_2 < 8 kpa (60 mm Hg) Irrespective of treatment with oxygen
- A low pH (or high H^+)

Caution: Patients with severe or life threatening attacks may not be distressed and may not have all these abnormalities. The presence of any should alert the doctor.

Near fatal asthma

- Raised $PaCO_2$
- Requiring IPPV with raised inflation pressures

IMMEDIATE TREATMENT

- Oxygen 40-60% (CO_2 retention is not usually aggravated by oxygen therapy in asthma)
- Salbutamol 5 mg or terbutaline 10 mg via an oxygen driven nebuliser
- Ipratropium bromide 0.5 mg via an oxygen driven nebuliser
- Prednisolone tablets 40-50 mg or IV hydrocortisone 100 mg or both if very ill
- No sedatives of any kind
- Chest radiograph only if pneumothorax or consolidation are suspected or patient requires IPPV

IF LIFE THREATENING FEATURES ARE PRESENT:

- Discuss with senior clinician and ICU team
- Add IV magnesium sulphate 1.2-2 g infusion over 20 minutes (unless already given)
- Give nebulised β_2 agonist more frequently e.g. salbutamol 5 mg up to every 15-30 minutes or 10 mg continuously hourly

SUBSEQUENT MANAGEMENT

IF PATIENT IS IMPROVING continue:
- 40-60% oxygen
- Prednisolone 40-50 mg daily or IV hydrocortisone 100 mg 6 hourly
- Nebulised β_2 agonist and ipratropium 4-6 hourly

IF PATIENT NOT IMPROVING AFTER 15-30 MINUTES:
- Continue oxygen and steroids
- Give nebulised β_2 agonist more frequently e.g. salbutamol 5 mg up to every 15-30 minutes or 10 mg continuously hourly
- Continue ipratropium 0.5 mg 4-6 hourly until patient is improving

IF PATIENT IS STILL NOT IMPROVING
- Discuss patient with senior clinician and ICU team
- IV magnesium sulphate 1.2-2 g over 20 minutes (unless already given)
- Senior clinician may consider use of IV β_2 agonist or IV aminophylline or progression to IPPV

Figure 4.2 Hospital management of acute severe asthma in adults, from the British Thoracic Society/Scottish Intercollegiate Guidelines Network (BTS/SIGN) asthma management guideline.[2] (Reproduced with permission from the BMJ Publishing Group.)

Management of acute severe asthma in adults in hospital

Peak expiratory flow in normal adults

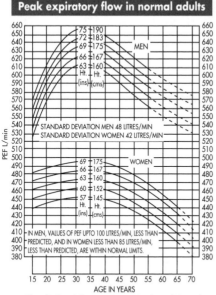

STANDARD DEVIATION MEN 48 LITRES/MIN
STANDARD DEVIATION WOMEN 42 LITRES/MIN

IN MEN, VALUES OF PEF UPTO 100 LITRES/MIN, LESS THAN
PREDICTED, AND IN WOMEN LESS THAN 85 LITRES/MIN,
LESS THAN PREDICTED, ARE WITHIN NORMAL LIMITS.

AGE IN YEARS

Nunn AJ, Gregg I. New regression equations for predicting peak
expiratory flow in adults, BMJ 1989;298:1068-70.

MONITORING

- Repeat measurement of PEF 15-30 minutes after starting treatment
- Oximetry: maintain $SpO_2 > 92\%$
- Repeat blood gas measurements within 2 hours of starting treatment if:
  - initial $PaO_2 < 8$ kPa (60 mm Hg) unless subsequent $SpO_2 > 92\%$
  - $PaCO_2$ normal or raised
  - Patient deteriorates
- Chart PEF before and after giving β_2 agonists and at least 4 times daily throughout hospital stay

Transfer to ICU accompanied by a doctor prepared to intubate if:

- Deteriorating PEF, worsening or persisting hypoxia, or hypercapnea
- Exhaustion, feeble respirations, confusion or drowsiness
- Coma or respiratory arrest

DISCHARGE

When discharged from hospital patients should have:

- Been on discharge medication for 24 hours and have had inhaler technique checked and recorded
- PEF > 75% of best or predicted and PEF diurnal variability < 25% unless discharge is agreed with respiratory physician
- Treatment with oral and inhaled steroids in addition to bronchodilators
- Own PEF meter and written asthma action plan
- GP follow up arranged within 2 working days
- Follow up appointment in respiratory clinic within 4 weeks

Patients with severe asthma (indicated by need for admission) and adverse behavioural or psychosocial features are at risk of further severe or fatal attacks

- Determine reason(s) for exacerbation and admission
- Send details of admission, discharge and potential best PEF to GP.

Figure 4.2   *continued*

Table 4.1 Prescribing of beta-2 agonists in adults, children and infants with acute asthma exacerbations

	Adults and children over 12 years of age	Children aged 2–12 years	Infants (under 2 years of age)
First-line treatment	Yes	Yes	Consider a trial
Method of administration	*Mild/moderate*: MDI plus spacer device *Severe*: as above or via nebuliser *Life-threatening*: nebuliser driven by oxygen.	*Mild/moderate*: MDI plus spacer device (children under 3 years are likely to require a facemask connected to the mouthpiece of a spacer) *Severe*: as above or via nebuliser *Life-threatening*: Nebuliser driven by oxygen	*Mild/moderate*: MDI plus spacer and close fitting facemask – as effective if not better than nebulisers for treating mild-to-moderate asthma *Severe*: via nebuliser *Life-threatening*: nebuliser driven by oxygen
Dosage	*Mild/moderate*: salbutamol, 200 micrograms, or terbutaline, 500 micrograms PRN *Severe/life-threatening*: Initially salbutamol, 5 mg, or terbutaline, 10 mg, nebulised. If the patient is improving, consider salbutamol 2.5 mg, 4–6 hourly or PRN. If the patient is not improving, give beta-2 agonist more frequently (e.g. salbutamol, 5 mg, up to every 10–15 minutes or continuous nebulisation (e.g. salbutamol, 5–10 mg/hour).	*Mild*: Salbutamol 200–400 micrograms (2–4 puffs), via spacer plus facemask, repeated every 20–30 minutes according to clinical response. Increase dose by 200 micrograms (2 puffs) every 2 minutes up to 1 mg (10 puffs) according to response. If good response, continue up to 10 puffs PRN (not exceeding 4 hourly). *Severe*: 1 mg (10 puffs) repeated according to clinical response. Consider nebulised administration. *Life-threatening*: nebulised salbutamol, 2.5 mg, or terbutaline, 5 mg ,with oxygen as driving gas. If life-threatening features present, repeat nebulised beta-2 agonist plus bolus intravenous salbutamol, 15 micrograms/kg, of 200 micrograms/ml solution over 10 minutes. Doses above 1–2 micrograms/kg/minute should be given in a paediatric intensive care unit.	*Mild/moderate*: Salbutamol up to 1 mg (10 puffs) via spacer and facemask *Severe/life-threatening*: MDI plus spacer ineffective. Nebulised salbutamol, 2.5 mg, or nebulised terbutaline, 5 mg. Repeated according to clinical response.

MDI, metered dose inhaler; PRN, *pro re nata* (as needed).

possible that there may be an advantage in higher doses in patients with the most severe obstruction. In practice, the acute episode should be efficiently controlled using high doses of beta-2 agonists. However, subsequent dose and dosing interval should be individualised using objective measures of lung function as a guide.

4. *Continuous versus intermittent nebulisation.* Continuous nebulisation is thought to be more beneficial than intermittent therapy; however, a meta-analysis of randomised controlled trials of adults with acute asthma found no significant differences between the two methods in terms of improvement in pulmonary function or hospital admission; nevertheless, continuous nebulisation was associated with fewer side-effects.[19] Most patients with acute asthma respond adequately to bolus nebulisation of beta-2 agonists.[3] The BTS/SIGN asthma management guideline recommends that continuous nebulisation (salbutamol, 5–10 mg/hour) should be considered in severe asthma (peak expiratory flow [PEF] or forced expiratory volume in 1 second [FEV_1] less than 50% best or predicted) and asthma that is poorly responsive to an initial dose of a beta-2 agonist.

Corticosteroids[3]

Systemic steroids should be given in adequate doses to all patients with acute asthma. Corticosteroids are not bronchodilators but are extremely effective in reducing the airway inflammation present in virtually all patients with asthma. They reduce mortality, relapses, subsequent hospital admission and requirement for beta-2 agonists. The earlier corticosteroids are given in an acute attack, the better the outcome. Steroid tablets are as effective as parenteral steroids, provided the tablets can be swallowed and retained and there is no problem with absorption. A soluble preparation is available for those unable to swallow tablets. A 5 day course of prednisolone, 40–50 mg daily, is recommended, although in practice the duration of treatment should be adjusted to bring about recovery.

Steroid tablets can be stopped abruptly after recovery from the acute exacerbation; there is no need to taper the dose of steroid, except in rare cases where the patient was previously on a maintenance dose of steroid or the steroid course was longer than 3 weeks.

Inhaled steroids do not provide additional benefit to the management of acute asthma but should be started as soon as possible or continued to be prescribed to ensure that the long-term management plan is adhered to (see Chapter 3).

Ipratropium bromide[3]

The use of inhaled ipratropium bromide as the initial bronchodilator for adults with acute asthma has been consistently reported to be inferior to the use of beta-2 agonists in improving airflow. However, the existing literature suggests that inhaled anticholinergic agents provide an additional benefit to children and adults with acute asthma who are treated with beta-2 agonists, with minimal side-effects. Ipratropium bromide should be added to nebulised beta-2 agonist treatment for patients with acute severe or life-threatening symptoms and for patients who show a poor response to administration of beta-2 agonist alone. The recommended dose in adults with acute asthma is 500 micrograms every 4–6 hours, reducing the frequency as clinical improvement occurs. The continued prescribing of ipratropium bromide once the condition is stable is not beneficial. Special caution is needed to protect the patient's eyes from the nebulised drug, as it has been reported to cause acute-angle glaucoma (see Chapter 11).

Intravenous magnesium

Magnesium is an intracellular ion that is essential for a wide range of cellular functions, including inhibition of calcium channels. It relaxes smooth muscle *in vitro* and is a weak bronchodilator but probably does not inhibit airway hyperresponsiveness.[21,22] The idea of using intravenous magnesium in asthma was first reported in 1936. A number of case reports and studies have reported on the role of intravenous magnesium given as a bolus (1.2–2 g over 20 minutes) in the management of acute severe asthma. A systematic review of the literature reported that, overall, there was no significant improvement in either hospital admissions or lung function, although there was a significant improvement in a subgroup analysis of more severely affected patients.[23] Another study showed that magnesium benefited a subgroup of patients presenting to the emergency department with an FEV_1 below 25%, further supporting the idea that magnesium should be administered to patients with life-threatening or near-fatal asthma,[24] which is the recommendation of the BTS/SIGN asthma management guideline.[2] The guideline also suggests that a single dose of intravenous magnesium be considered for patients with acute severe asthma who have not had a good initial response to inhaled bronchodilator therapy. The *Drugs and Therapeutics Bulletin* recently reviewed the evidence for administration of intravenous magnesium in acute severe asthma and, contrary to the recent BTS/SIGN guideline, concluded that the evidence "is weak and conflicting and does not justify the unlicensed use of this drug."[25]

Intravenous aminophylline

The role of aminophylline in the treatment of severe acute asthma has been challenged since the advent of potent selective beta-2 agonists. At therapeutic doses, aminophylline is a weaker bronchodilator than the beta-2 agonists, and it has many undesirable side-effects. Furthermore, intravenous aminophylline may not provide any additional benefit when administered to patients already receiving beta-2 agonists and corticosteroids. The BTS/SIGN asthma management guideline therefore does not recommend the routine use of intravenous aminophylline in the treatment of acute asthma. If the response to standard treatment is poor, individual patients with life-threatening asthma may benefit from intravenous aminophylline. In these cases, a loading dose of 5 mg/kg over 20 minutes (unless on maintenance oral therapy, when no loading dose is given) followed by an infusion of 500–700 micrograms/kg/hour; daily measurement of blood theophylline levels is recommended.

Leukotriene receptor antagonists

Data on the effects of leukotriene receptor antagonists in acute asthma are limited and they are therefore not recommended for managing acute asthma.

Antibiotics

Antibiotics are not an effective treatment for acute asthma, as infections that precipitate an acute attack are usually viral. Routine prescription of antibiotics for all patients with acute asthma is not indicated.[2]

Heliox

The administration of heliox, a helium–oxygen mixture, reduces turbulent airflow across narrowed airways, which can help to reduce the work of breathing. This, in turn, can improve gas exchange, arterial blood gas levels and clinical symptoms. Some data suggest that nebulised-size particles may be distributed more uniformly in the distal airways when nebulisation treatments are administered via heliox than with a standard oxygen–nitrogen mixture. The effectiveness of heliox in reducing the density of administered gas and improving laminar airflow depends on the helium concentration of the gas – the higher the helium concentration, the more effective the result; an 80:20 mixture of helium–oxygen is most effective. However, the current evidence is not sufficient to establish the administration of heliox in routine care.[2]

Other therapies

Inhaled anaesthetic agents (e.g. halothane, isoflurane and enflurane) have been used with varying degrees of success in intubated patients with refractory severe asthma. The mechanism of action is unclear but they may have direct relaxant effects on airway smooth muscle.

Additional management options

Some case reports describe successful use of extracorporeal membrane oxygenation in extreme cases of refractory status asthmaticus in which maximum standard pharmacotherapy and mechanical ventilation was unsuccessful.

Ventilatory assistance can be life saving, and both non-invasive and invasive techniques are available. The decision to intubate a patient with asthma is taken with extreme caution. Positive-pressure ventilation in a patient with asthma is complicated by severe airways obstruction and air trapping, resulting in hyperinflated lungs that may resist further inflation, placing the patient at high risk of barotrauma. Therefore, mechanical ventilation should be undertaken only in the face of continued deterioration despite maximal bronchodilatory therapy. Non-invasive facemask ventilation may offer short-term support for some patients with hypercapnic respiratory failure who are gradually tiring and can cooperate with their care. It is not recommended for use in the place of mechanical ventilation in cases of very acute asthma, as further studies are required.

Management of acute asthma in children

The principles of treating acute asthma in children are the same as in adults but there are differences in dosages of medication and clinical assessment (Figure 4.3).

Management of acute asthma in children in hospital

Age 2-5 years

ASSESS ASTHMA SEVERITY

Moderate exacerbation
- SpO₂ ≥ 92%
- No clinical features of severe asthma

NB: If a patient has signs and symptoms across categories, always treat according to their most severe features

Severe exacerbation
- SpO₂ < 92%
- Too breathless to talk or eat
- Heart rate > 130/min
- Respiratory rate > 50/min
- Use of accessory neck muscles

Life threatening asthma
- SpO₂ < 92%
- Silent chest
- Poor respiratory effort
- Agitation
- Altered consciousness
- Cyanosis

Oxygen via face masks/nasal prongs to achieve normal saturations

Moderate:
- β₂ agonist 2-4 puffs via spacer ± face mask
- Increase β₂ agonist dose by 2 puffs every 2 minutes up to 10 puffs according to response
- Consider soluble oral prednisolone 20 mg

Reassess within 1 hour

Severe:
- β₂ agonist 10 puffs via spacer ± face mask or nebulised salbutamol 2.5 mg or terbutaline 5 mg
- Soluble prednisolone 20 mg or IV hydrocortisone 4 mg/kg
- Repeat β₂ agonist up to every 20-30 minutes according to response
- If poor response add 0.25 mg nebulised ipratropium bromide

Life threatening:
- Nebulised β₂ agonist salbutamol 2.5 mg or terbutaline 5 mg plus ipratropium bromide 0.25 mg nebulised
- IV hydrocortisone 4 mg/kg

Discuss with senior clinician, PICU team or paediatrician

- Repeat bronchodilators every 20-30 minutes

ASSESS RESPONSE TO TREATMENT
Record respiratory rate, heart rate and oxygen saturation every 1-4 hours

RESPONDING
- Continue bronchodilators 1-4 hours prn
- Discharge when stable on 4 hourly treatment
- Continue oral prednisolone for up to 3 days

At discharge
- Ensure stable on 4 hourly inhaled treatment and
- Review the need for regular treatment and the use of inhaled steroids
- Review inhaler technique
- Provide a written asthma action plan for treating future attacks
- Arrange follow up according to local policy

NOT RESPONDING
- Arrange HDU/PICU transfer
Consider:
- Chest x-ray and blood gases
- IV salbutamol 15 mcg/kg bolus over 10 minutes followed by continuous infusion 1-5 mcg/kg/min (dilute to 200 mcg/ml)
- IV aminophylline 5 mg/kg loading dose over 20 minutes (omit in those receiving oral theophyllines) followed by continuous infusion 1 mg/kg/hour

Age >5 years

ASSESS ASTHMA SEVERITY

Moderate exacerbation
- SpO₂ ≥ 92%
- PEF ≥ 50% best or predicted
- No clinical features of severe asthma

NB: If a patient has signs and symptoms across categories, always treat according to their most severe features

Severe exacerbation
- SpO₂ < 92%
- PEF < 50% best or predicted
- Heart rate > 120/min
- Respiratory rate > 30/min
- Use of accessory neck muscles

Life threatening asthma
- SpO₂ < 92%
- PEF < 33% best or predicted
- Silent chest
- Poor respiratory effort
- Altered consciousness
- Cyanosis

Oxygen via face masks/nasal prongs to achieve normal saturations

Moderate:
- β₂ agonist 2-4 puffs via spacer
- Increase β₂ agonist dose by 2 puffs every 2 minutes up to 10 puffs according to response
- Oral prednisolone 30-40 mg

Reassess within 1 hour

Severe:
- β₂ agonist 10 puffs via spacer or nebulised salbutamol 2.5-5 mg or terbutaline 5-10 mg
- Oral prednisolone 30-40 mg or IV hydrocortisone 4 mg/kg if vomiting
- If poor response nebulised ipratropium bromide 0.25 mg
- Repeat β₂ agonist and ipratropium up to every 20-30 minutes according to response

Life threatening:
- Nebulised β₂ agonist salbutamol 5 mg or terbutaline 10 mg plus ipratropium bromide 0.25 mg nebulised
- IV hydrocortisone 4 mg/kg

Discuss with senior clinician, PICU team and paediatrician

- Repeat bronchodilators every 20-30 minutes

ASSESS RESPONSE TO TREATMENT
Record respiratory rate, heart rate and oxygen saturation and PEF/FEV every 1-4 hours

RESPONDING
- Continue bronchodilators 1-4 hours pm
- Discharge when stable on 4 hourly treatment
- Continue oral prednisolone 30-40 mg for up to 3 days

At discharge
- Ensure stable on 4 hourly inhaled treatment
- Review the need for regular treatment and
- Review inhaler technique
- Provide a written asthma action plan for treating future attacks
- Arrange follow up according to local policy

NOT RESPONDING
- Continue 20-30 minutes nebulisers and arrange HDU/PICU transfer
Consider:
- Chest x-ray and blood gases
- Bolus IV salbutamol 15 mcg/kg if not already given
- Continuous IV salbutamol infusion 1-5 mcg/kg/min (200 mcg/ml solution)
- IV aminophylline 5 mg/kg loading dose over 20 minutes followed by continuous infusion 1 mg/kg/hour (omit in those receiving oral theophylline)
- Bolus IV infusion of magnesium sulphate 40 mg/kg (max 2 g over 20 minutes)

Figure 4.3 Hospital management of acute asthma in children, from the British Thoracic Society/Scottish Intercollegiate Guidelines Network (BTS/SIGN) asthma management guideline.[2] (Reproduced with permission from the BMJ Publishing Group.)

Treatment of acute asthma in children over 2 years of age

Beta-2 agonists

In children (2–12 years of age), beta-2 agonists are superior to all other bronchodilators since they work effectively within minutes of adminis-tration and should be administered as first-line therapy, usually by inhalation. An MDI with a spacer device provides an effective way to administer the beta-2 agonist to children with mild-to-moderate asthma and is less likely to induce tachycardia and hypoxia than when the same drug is given via a nebuliser.[26] Children under 3 years of age are likely to require a facemask connected to the mouthpiece of the spacer device to aid successful drug delivery. It is important that the facemask fits tightly, as inhalation through a facemask 2–3 cm from the face will reduce drug delivery by as much as 85%.[27] The dose of inhaled beta-2 agonist required to treat acute asthma in children depends on the severity of the disease and should be adjusted according to the patient's response. For mild asthma exacerbations, 2–4 puffs (i.e. 200–400 micrograms salbutamol) repeated every 20–30 minutes might be sufficient, whereas up to 10 puffs may be required in a severe attack. Continuous nebulised beta-2 agonists are of no greater benefit than frequent as-required doses in the same total hourly dosage.[28,29] The role of intravenous beta-2 agonists in children remains unclear.

For children with severe acute asthma or in those where there is uncertainty about reliable drug delivery via the inhalation route, the recommendation is to either add a bolus dose of intravenous salbuta-mol (15 micrograms/kg) to maximal doses of nebulised salbutamol or to start a continuous intravenous infusion.

Corticosteroids

Steroids should be administered as early as possible after initial presentation – prednisolone, 20 mg daily, for children aged 2–5 years; 30–40 mg daily for children over 5 years of age. Oral administration is effective in the majority of children. A soluble preparation can be used for those unable to swallow tablets. Parenteral administration is recom-mended only if the child is unable to retain oral medication. The inhaled route is not recommended for the treatment of acute symptoms but children who are already using inhaled corticosteroids should continue with their usual maintenance dose. There is insufficient evidence to support increasing the dose of inhaled steroid in an exacerbation. Treat-ment with oral prednisolone for 3 days is usually sufficient but the length of course should be tailored to the individual and continued until recovery.[2]

Anticholinergics

Anticholinergics, such as ipratropium, are recommended for children who respond poorly to beta-2 agonists. Administered alone, ipratropium has no role in the management of acute severe asthma in this age group. However, the combination of a beta-2 agonist and an anticholinergic produces better results than either drug used alone and benefits are more apparent in severe cases. Frequent doses (250 micrograms /dose nebulised up to every 20–30 minutes) should be used in the initial stages of an asthma attack. The dose frequency should be reduced as clinical improvement occurs.

Intravenous aminophylline

As in adults with acute asthma, intravenous aminophylline is not recommended in children with mild-to-moderate acute asthma but should be considered for children with severe or life-threatening bronchospasm that is unresponsive to maximal doses of bronchodilators and steroid tablets.

Other therapies

There is no evidence to support the use of heliox, leukotriene antagonists or routine antibiotics for the treatment of acute asthma in children. Intravenous magnesium is a safe treatment although its place in therapy is not yet established.

Treatment of acute asthma in children under 2 years of age

Management of acute asthma attacks in children under 2 years of age is complicated by differences in lung anatomy and physiology compared with older children and a poorer response to treatments. Several early studies showed no bronchodilator response to beta-2 agonists in children under 2 years of age with asthma, encouraging the debate that infants do not have functioning beta-2–receptors from birth.[30–32] More recent studies have shown that beta-2–receptors are present and function from birth but that the response to beta-2–receptors can be small and there is marked inter-individual variation.[33,34] A trial of inhaled beta-2 agonist is recommended for the initial treatment of acute asthma.[2] For mild-to-moderate acute asthma, an MDI with a spacer device and mask is the preferred method of drug delivery, although a nebuliser can be used if there is doubt or concern about effective drug delivery.

Oral corticosteroid tablets (e.g. 10 mg soluble prednisolone daily for up to 3 days) should be started as early as possible and used in conjunction with beta-2 agonists.[2]

In severe cases, the addition of ipratropium bromide to the beta-2 agonists and corticosteroids may produce some improvement in clinical symptoms and reduce the need for more intensive treatment.[2]

Discharge from hospital after an acute attack

A patient can be discharged from hospital when they have recovered sufficiently from an acute attack. There should be good air entry without wheezing and the PEF should be greater than 75% predicted or personal best. Oxygen saturation should be greater than 92% (94% for children) when breathing room air. The patient's requirement for beta-2 agonists should be decreasing and preferably no more than every 4 hours, and they should be taking medication that could easily be continued safely at home.

An acute exacerbation of asthma should be regarded as a failure of long-term asthma care, and ways of helping patients and families to avoid further severe episodes should be considered. The discharge plan should address the following points.

- Check the patient's inhaler technique.
- Consider the need for regular inhaled corticosteroids.
- Provide a written action plan (see Chapter 8).
- Ensure the patient has a full understanding of medications to be taken.
- Ensure the patient is followed up by their general practitioner within 1 week (children) or 2 days (adults).
- Ensure the patient is followed up by a hospital physician within 1–2 months (children) or 1 month (adults).

References

1. The Burden of Lung Disease: A statistics report from the British Thoracic Society, 2001 *www.brit-thoracic.co.uk*
2. British Thoracic Society/Scottish Intercollegiate Guidelines Network. British Guideline on the Management of Asthma. *Thorax* 2003; 58 (Suppl I): S1–S94.

3. Rodrigo GJ, Rodrigo C, Hall JB. Acute asthma in adults: a review. *Chest* 2004; 125: 1081–1102.

4. Turner MO, Noertjojo K, Vedal S, *et al*. Risk factors for near-fatal asthma: a case-control study in hospitalized patients with asthma. *Am J Respir Crit Care Med* 1998; 157: 1804–1809.

5. Hessel PA, Mitchell I, Tough S, *et al*. Risk factors for death from asthma. *Ann Allergy Asthma Immunol* 1999; 83: 362–368.

6. Abramson MJ, Bailey MJ, Couper FJ, *et al*. Are asthma medications and management related to deaths from asthma? *Am J Respir Crit Care Med* 2001; 163: 12–18.

7. Plaza V, Serrano J, Picado C, *et al*. Frequency and clinical characteristics of rapid-onset fatal and near-fatal asthma. *Eur Respir J* 2002; 19: 846–852.

8. Carroll N, Carello S, Cooke C, James A. Airway structure and inflammatory cells in fatal attacks of asthma. *Eur Respir J* 1996; 9: 709–715.

9. Carroll N, Elliot J, Motron A, James A. The structure of large and small airways in nonfatal and fatal asthma. *Am Rev Respir Dis* 1993; 147: 405–410.

10. Dales RE, Cakmak S, Judek S, *et al*. The role of fungal spores in thunderstorm asthma. *Chest* 2003; 123: 745–750.

11. Marks GB, Colquhoun JR, Girgis ST, *et al*. Thunderstorm outflows preceding epidemics of asthma during spring and summer. *Thorax* 2001; 56: 468–471.

12. Packe GE, Ayres JG. Asthma outbreak during a thunderstorm. *Lancet* 1985; 2: 199–204

13. Higham J, Venables K, Kopek E, *et al*. Asthma and thunderstorms: description of an epidemic in general practice in Britain using data from a doctors' deputising service in the UK. *J Epidemiol Commun Health* 1997; 51: 233–238.

14. Venables KM, Allitt U, Collier CG, *et al*. Thunderstorm-related asthma: the epidemic of 24/25 June 1994. *Clin Exp Allergy* 1997; 27: 725–736.

15. Celenza A, Fothergill J, Kupek E, *et al*. Thunderstorm associated asthma: a detailed analysis of environmental factors. *BMJ* 1996; 312: 604–607.

16. McFadden ER. Acute severe asthma. *Am J Resp Crit Care Med* 2003; 168: 740–759.

17. Travers A, Jones AP, Kelly K, *et al*. Intravenous beta-2 agonists for acute asthma in the emergency department (Cochrane Review) In: *The Cochrane Library*, issue 3. Chichester: John Wiley & Sons, 2001 (*www.thecochrane library.com*).

18. Bradding P, Rushby I, Scullion J, *et al*. As required versus regular nebulised salbutamol for the treatment of acute severe asthma. *Eur Respir J* 1999; 13: 290–294.

19. Emerman CL, Cydulka RK, McFadden ER. Comparison of 2.5 mg versus 7.5 mg of inhaled albuterol in the treatment of acute asthma. *Chest* 1999; 115: 92–96.

20. Rodrigo GJ, Rodrigo C. Continuous vs intermittent beta-2 agonists in the treatment of acute adult asthma: a systematic review with meta-analysis. *Chest* 2002; 122: 160–165.

21. Hill JM, Britton J. Effect of intravenous magnesium sulphate on airway calibre

and airway reactivity to histamine in asthmatic subjects. *Br J Clin Pharmacol* 1996; 42: 629–631.

22. Hill J, Lewis S, Britton J. Studies of the effects of inhaled magnesium on airway reactivity to histamine and adenosine monophosphate in asthmatic subjects. *Clin Exp Allergy* 1997; 27: 546–551.

23. Rowe BH, Bretzlaff JA, Bourdon C, *et al*. Intravenous magnesium sulfate treatment for acute asthma in the emergency department: a systematic review of the literature. *Ann Emerg Med* 2000; 36: 181–190.

24. Silverman RA, Osborn H, Runge J, *et al*. IV magnesium sulfate in the treatment of acute severe asthma: a multicenter randomized controlled trial. *Chest* 2002; 122: 489–497.

25. Anonymous. Intravenous magnesium for acute asthma. *Drugs Ther Bull* 2003; 41: 79–80.

26. Cates CJ, Rowe BH, Bara A. Holding chambers versus nebulisers for beta-agonist treatment of acute asthma (Cochrane Review). *The Cochrane Library*, issue 3. Chichester: John Wiley & Sons, 2001 (*www.thecochranelibrary.com*).

27. Everard ML, Clark AR, Milner AD. Drug delivery from holding chambers with attached facemask. *Arch Dis Child* 1992; 67: 580–585.

28. Khine H, Fuchs SM, Saville AL. Continuous vs intermittent nebulised albuterol for emergency management of asthma. *Acad Emerg Med* 1996; 3: 1019–1024.

29. Papo MC, Frank J, Thompson AE. A prospective, randomized study of continuous versus intermittent nebulised albuterol for severe status asthmaticus in children. *Crit Care Med* 1993; 21: 1479–1486.

30. Lenney W, Milner AD. At what age do bronchodilator drugs work? *Arch Dis Child* 1978; 53: 532–535.

31. Lenney W, Evans NAP. Nebulised salbutamol and ipratropium bromide in asthmatic children. *Br J Dis Chest* 1986; 80: 59–65.

32. Chavasse RJ, Bastian-Lee Y, Richter H, *et al*. Inhaled salbutamol for wheezy infants: a randomised controlled trial. *Arch Dis Child* 2000; 82: 370–375.

33. Yuksel B, Greenough A. Effect of nebulised salbutamol in preterm infants during the first year of life. *Eur Respir J* 1991; 4: 1088–1092.

34. Wilkie RA, Bryan MH. Effect of bronchodilator on airway resistance in ventilator-dependent neonates with chronic lung disease. *J Paediatr* 1987; 111: 278–282.

5

Lifestyle management

The successful treatment of asthma depends to a large degree on motivating the patient to take responsibility for the day-to-day management of their condition. Key to this is providing the patient with a good understanding of the nature of asthma and its treatment. Patients need to understand that there is no cure for asthma but there is excellent treatment that can allow virtually anyone with asthma to lead a normal life. Although much of the management of asthma is pharmacologically based, special attention should be given to lifestyle modifications, such as avoiding exposure to factors that worsen asthma, enabling the patient to manage their condition and to maintain an active and independent lifestyle.

Allergen avoidance

Approximately 80% of children and 50% of adults with asthma are atopic.[1] For these individuals, exposure to allergens is associated with increased asthma symptoms, bronchial reactivity and deterioration in lung function.[2] Exposure to high concentrations of indoor allergens can increase requirement for treatment and may lead to hospital admission and respiratory arrest. Many different allergens can cause sensitivity; however, a large proportion of atopic individuals are sensitive to house dust mite or animal allergens, particularly cat and dog dander.

House dust mite

The house dust mite *Dermatophagoides pteronyssinus* is a microscopic invertebrate. The mites feed off the tiny particles of skin that are constantly shed by people and animals. While the mite itself contains some allergens, the real problem is with its faeces, which float in the air and accumulate in many areas around the house, particularly bedding, carpets and upholstered furniture.

Evidence for the efficacy of allergen control measures in the domestic environment as prophylaxis of asthma is conflicting. A large number of strategies can be used in an attempt to eradicate dust mites but in reality it is difficult in normal homes to substantially reduce the level of allergen. It has been shown that moving mite-sensitive patients with asthma to low-allergen environments, such as allergen-free hospital rooms or high-altitude sanatoriums, reduces airway reactivity and inflammation,[3,4] although these improvements might be a result of factors other than the low-allergen environment.

Two Cochrane reviews have looked at house dust mite control measures and the management of asthma.[5,6] Recommendations to go to great lengths to eradicate house dust mites are based on the assumption that, because house dust mites trigger asthma attacks, fewer mites should lead to fewer asthma attacks. However, the Cochrane review of trials was unable to confirm this. The first review concluded that people with asthma did not experience a significant reduction in the number or severity of asthma exacerbations after increased physical house cleaning and use of chemical methods against dust mites. The second review amended these findings, and concluded that physical methods may have some effect. The Cochrane reviewers suggested several theories to explain the lack of impact of anti-dust-mite activities in the trials.

- Patients may find it difficult to adhere to the vigorous cleaning procedures required in the trials.
- The population of mites may not have been reduced enough to make a difference to the individual's asthma exacerbations.
- Patients may also be allergic to other allergens within the house, which could continue to trigger asthma exacerbations, even when there are fewer house dust mites.

Importantly, the Cochrane reviewers pointed out flaws in the research. There was heterogeneity between studies with regard to intervention, and in some studies intervention allocation was not adequately concealed. Thus, larger and more carefully controlled studies are required to demonstrate any clear benefit from house dust mite avoidance and, at present, this does not appear to be a cost-effective method of achieving benefit. The British Thoracic Society Guidelines/Scottish Intercollegiate Guidelines Network (BTS/SIGN)[2] asthma management guideline recommends a number of measures in committed families with evidence of house dust mite allergy and who wish to try mite avoidance, described in the Management Focus on page 83.

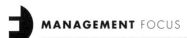

> **Advice for avoiding house dust mite, from the British Thoracic Society/Scottish Intercollegiate Guidelines Network (BTS/SIGN) asthma management guideline[2]**
>
> - Use complete barrier bed-covering systems
> - Remove carpets
> - Remove soft toys from beds
> - Wash bed linen at high temperature
> - Apply acaricides to soft furnishings
> - Use dehumidifiers

Some strategies, such as avoiding feather bedding, might in fact be counter-productive. Bedding often has high concentration of dust mites and many people have assumed that bedding made from feathers would gather more mites than bedding of synthetic (manmade) fibre. However, the Cochrane review found studies that show synthetic bedding can actually harbour more dust mites than the bedding made with feathers. Studies have also shown that people with asthma who used synthetic bedding had more asthma attacks than those whose bedding is made of feathers. However, these studies are not trials comparing one form of bedding with another, so they do not provide a reliable answer for people who want to know which bedding would be better for them; indeed, there are no trials that address this issue. There is no evidence that any cleaning routine for bedding makes a difference to the number of asthma attacks. Therefore, the common recommendations about bedding for people with asthma seem to be based more on convention than evidence. Personal trial and error may be the best guide.

Activities that claim to give patients control over their asthma might be welcome for some people, whereas for others some of these regimens will be unfeasible or too disruptive. Personal experience will guide people as to what is worthwhile in their lives

Other allergens

People can be allergic to various animals, including birds. An allergy to cats and dogs is common in people with asthma living in developed countries and it is undisputable that sensitisation to pets is an important risk factor for asthma. Patients with asthma who are pet sensitised and are exposed either to the pet or to high levels of pet allergen tend to have more severe symptoms than those who are not exposed. It is possible for patients to become sensitised to pets even if they have never lived with them. For people who are allergic to animals, the allergen is often the dander – scales that come off fur or feathers. However, people can be allergic to other substances coming from animals, such as gland secretions, saliva or substances in the urine. Observational studies have not found that removing a pet from a home improves asthma control.[7] Controversially, it has been suggested that maintaining a high exposure to cat allergen in the domestic environment might induce some degree of tolerance.[8] A Cochrane review is underway to determine whether measures to reduce pet allergens also reduce asthma severity. Although the evidence is inconclusive, many experts still feel that removal of pets from the home of individuals with asthma who also have an allergy to that pet should be recommended. For those who want to keep a family pet, some people recommend keeping the pet out of the bedroom, frequent washing of pets or air filtration, although there is no evidence to show that these strategies reduce asthma exacerbations.

Avoiding pollutants

Smoking

Twenty-seven per cent of the UK population smoke tobacco. There are at least as many active cigarette smokers amongst people with asthma as in the general population – studies have indicated that 20–35% of people with asthma are regular smokers.[9,10] There is evidence to indicate that asthma sufferers who smoke are at an increased risk of morbidity and mortality, including more severe symptoms, more severe exacerbations and more rapid decline in lung function.[11,12] The negative effects of smoking on asthma have been attributed to the observations that smoking can promote inflammation and remodelling of the airways. A further study suggests that smoking may also block the beneficial effects of corticosteroids. Although more evidence is required in this area,[13] if it proves to be true, asthmatics who smoke may be blocking the effects of the treatment that can prevent their asthma from deteriorating.

According to a *No Smoking Day* survey in 2002, 72% of smokers would like to give up.[14] Smoking cessation should be encouraged, as it is good for general health and may decrease asthma severity. The Health Education Authority published smoking cessation guidelines for health professionals in the journal *Thorax* in 1998 and updated them in 2000.[15] The guidelines are known as the 'five As': **Ask, Advise, Assess,**

Assist, Arrange. The Royal College of Nursing's tobacco education project flowchart shows how to put these guidelines into daily practice (see Figure 5.1).

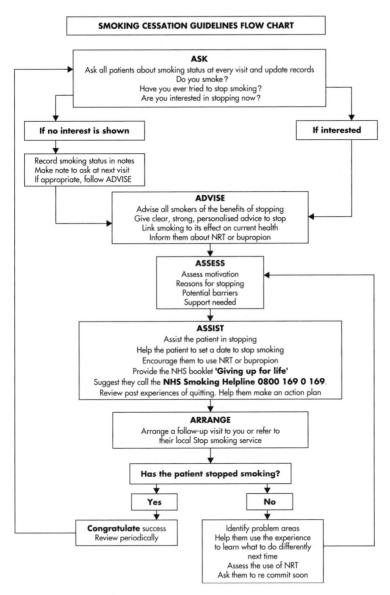

Figure 5.1   The Royal College of Nursing smoking cessation guidelines flowchart. (Reproduced with permission of the Royal College of Nursing Tobacco Education Project; Percival J. *Clearing The Air 2, Smoking And Tobacco Control – An Updated Guide For Nurses.* London: RCN, 2000.) NRT, nicotine-replacement therapy.

The National Institute for Health and Clinical Excellence (NICE) has produced guidance on nicotine replacement therapy (NRT) and bupropion hydrochloride (Zyban) after evaluating their clinical effectiveness.[16] The NICE guideline recommends that both products should be available on NHS prescription for smokers who express a desire to quit smoking, and highlighted that providing advice and support was of major importance. It was suggested that the initial NRT prescription should be sufficient to last 2 weeks from the quit date, with further prescriptions given as the quit attempt continues successfully. NICE also stated that prescribing NRT or bupropion hydrochloride was amongst the most cost-effective of all healthcare interventions.

Air pollution

There is evidence that changing from a high-particulate sulphur dioxide (coal-burning) environment to a low-sulphur-dioxide/high-diesel particulate environment increases the incidence of asthma and atopy.[1] In the UK, asthma is more prevalent in 12–14 year olds in non-metropolitan rather than metropolitan areas. However, there are many differences between the two environments that may explain the variation in asthma risk. Studies have shown that air pollution may provoke acute asthma attacks or aggravate existing chronic asthma. Fluctuations in air pollution may explain small changes in the number of hospital admissions and attendances at emergency departments for asthma.[17]

Complementary therapies/alternative medicines

Breathing techniques

People with asthma are increasingly using breathing techniques to manage their disease. A recent patient survey by Asthma UK (formerly the National Asthma Campaign) found that 30% of responders reported using breathing techniques for asthma control.[18] Unfortunately, the current evidence base for the effectiveness of breathing techniques in asthma is inadequate to identify which techniques are effective and which patients may benefit.

Breathing techniques have been used to treat asthma in western society for many years, long before effective pharmacological medication were available. Techniques have generally focused on manipulating the respiratory pattern to reduce respiratory frequency and hyperventilation, and to encourage diaphragmatic breathing. Many different types of breathing techniques can be employed, for example yoga breathing exercises (pranayama), the Buteyko method, inspiratory muscle training and a physiotherapist-based breathing retraining programmes for hyperventilation.

The Buteyko method is probably one of the best-known breathing techniques for asthma after being the subject of a BBC *Panorama* television report and a series in the *Daily Telegraph*. The method, advocated by the Russian physician Konstantin Buteyko, is based on the belief that asthma is caused by hyperventilation and represents the body's homeostatic attempt to conserve carbon dioxide.[19] The breathing exercises concentrate on increasing the breath-holding time and on nasal breathing rather than mouth breathing. Patients' mouths are often taped closed over night to promote effective nasal breathing. Some reports have shown a reduction in bronchodilator use[20] and reported an improvement in asthma symptoms; however, well-designed clinical trials in this area are lacking.

Asthma is accepted as being an inflammatory disease of the airways. However, it is recognised that there is a poor correlation between airway obstruction and symptoms, with some patients having high symptom levels despite normal or near-normal lung function.[21] Hyperventilation and dysfunctional breathing patterns may in themselves result in symptoms that include breathlessness and chest tightness and so may overlap with the symptoms of asthma. Also, it has been shown that psychosocial and emotional factors may affect the patient's perception of their breathlessness, irrespective of asthma severity. Panic disorders and high anxiety levels are more common in people with asthma compared with the general population.[22] It is possible that for asthma patients who breathe abnormally, breathing techniques may improve outcomes through non-specific psychological mechanisms.

Herbal and traditional Chinese medicine

The evidence currently available to support the use of herbal or traditional Chinese medicines for the management of asthma is inconclusive.

Acupuncture

A number of clinical trials have investigated the benefit of acupuncture for the treatment of asthma. However, a Cochrane review raised many methodological concerns and found no evidence for a clinically valuable benefit from acupuncture. No statistical improvement in lung function could be demonstrated.[23]

Air ionisers

Air ionisers are frequently advertised and marketed as being beneficial to patients with asthma. Although they reduce levels of dust mite allergen in the room in which they are used, they have not been shown to have any effect on asthma symptoms or lung function. The BTS/SIGN asthma management guideline does not recommend the use of air ionisers to manage asthma.[2]

Homeopathy

The management of asthma with homeopathic medicines has been the subject of a Cochrane review.[24] The evidence is inconclusive and large well-designed clinical trials are required.

Some homeopaths and bee keepers suggest that people who have allergic reactions to pollens should eat local honey regularly in order to build up immunity to local pollens. However, there is no systematic review on this issue.

Hypnosis

Studies of hypnosis in the management people with asthma are generally flawed. Hypnosis may be effective, but more randomised and appropriately controlled studies are required.

Manual therapy

Manual therapy includes massage and spinal manipulation. Evidence from limited research indicates that there is no place for chiropractic in asthma management. No conclusions can be drawn on the use of massage techniques.

Dietary manipulation

Minerals

There is no direct evidence about the impact of salt in the diet of people with asthma although the incidence of asthma is higher in societies where salt is a more common part of the diet. A Cochrane review is looking at whether reducing salt in the diet can affect asthma.

Low ingestion of magnesium has been linked with a higher prevalence of asthma and an intervention study has suggested that magnesium supplementation reduces bronchial hyperresponsiveness and wheeze.[25] Other studies have investigated the effects of supplementing with sodium, selenium and vitamin C but have shown no benefit amongst patients with asthma.[2]

Fish oils and fatty acids

A Cochrane review concluded that there is little evidence in support of the recommendation to supplement the diet of people with asthma with fish oils (omega-3 fatty acids).[26]

Food additives

Artificial food additives are used in the mass production of many foods. Whether these can trigger asthma attacks is controversial, but it may be possible that food additives can trigger wheezing. The observed association between food additives and asthma is not a new one. Reports on children whose asthma appeared to be exacerbated by food colours date from 1958. Tartrazine (FDC yellow no. 5/E102) is one of the azo family of dyes and is a common colouring used in foods and drugs. The UK Government is encouraging manufacturers to remove such colourings from food products, particularly those aimed at school children. Tartrazine is banned in Norway and Finland.

Evidence as to whether tartrazine causes exacerbations of asthma is conflicting. Some studies found a positive association, particularly in individuals who are sensitive to aspirin whereas others have not demonstrated any link between tartrazine and asthma.[27] A Cochrane review reported that there is no evidence that tartrazine makes asthma worse or that avoiding it improves asthma symptoms. Routine exclusion of tartrazine from the diet may not benefit most patients, except the few individuals with proven sensitivity.[27]

Weight reduction in obese patients with asthma

A small randomised parallel-group study has shown improved asthma control following weight reduction in obese patients with asthma.[28] The BTS/SIGN asthma management guideline recommends that obese patients with asthma should be encouraged to lose weight, as it will improve their asthma symptoms.[2]

Exercise

Regular exercise can help improve asthma control. Avoiding exercise because of shortness of breath can lead to a dangerous spiral of inactivity (see Figure 5.2).

Although exercise may trigger some patient's asthma, this does not mean that they should stop taking any form of exercise. In fact, many sports stars, for example Paula Radcliffe, Ian Botham, Austin Healy and Ian Wright, have certainly not allowed asthma to affect their success. If their asthma is under control, the person should be able to enjoy any sport or exercise. Perhaps the only cautions are for sports such as scuba diving and sports when performed at high altitude such as climbing, hiking and skiing.

Patients may need to use a short-acting beta-2 agonist prophylactically about 15 minutes before starting to exercise and they should also be advised to keep the bronchodilator close at hand at all times. A warm-up session of 5–10 minutes can help to reduce exercise-induced breathlessness. Avoiding conditions that trigger the person's asthma may help, such as cold, dry days and high pollen counts. If an asthmatic patient becomes wheezy on exercise, it is a sign that their asthma may not be properly under control and their treatment may need to be adjusted.

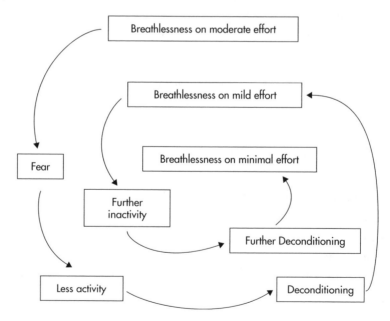

Figure 5.2 The spiral of inactivity.

Pulmonary rehabilitation

Pulmonary rehabilitation involves exercise training, counselling, education and dietetic input. Most patients who meet the criteria for a rehabilitation scheme will have chronic obstructive pulmonary disease; however, the benefits can apply to all patients with breathlessness, including those with chronic asthma. The exercise component of the programme is personalised to the patient's capabilities and individual goals. Current guidelines state that the exercise component of pulmonary rehabilitation should consist of aerobic (cardiovascular) exercises combined with exercises for the upper and lower limbs to achieve generalised strengthening of peripheral muscles. It is important to provide a home exercise programme.

Immunotherapy

Immunotherapy for allergies is highly controversial. Allergen immunotherapy – an attempt to 'immunise' a person against her or his own allergy – is also called hyposensitisation or desensitisation. Small but increasing amounts of the identified allergen are injected under the person's skin several times over weeks or months in an attempt to accustom the body to the allergen and hopefully neutralise the body's response to it. One of the main reasons for the controversy is that the injection can cause a severe reaction – even life-threatening anaphylaxis.

Immunotherapy injections (subcutaneous immunotherapy) have been available for some time. Other kinds of immunotherapy are also being developed, including tablets (to swallow or to hold under the tongue) and inhalants (to breathe in).

Clinical trials investigating immunotherapy for asthma have found positive results in certain patients, who demonstrate fewer asthma symptoms and reduced need for asthma medication. However, it is not known how this compares with other asthma treatments and further comparative studies are required.[2]

Travel

A small number of people with severe asthma may have difficulties with travelling although this can be overcome with determination and good medical advice. Travel within the UK is usually not a problem but air travel may present more difficulties. All people with severe asthma (or if they are concerned) should check with their doctor before planning a holiday, especially if they want to fly or travel abroad. As long as the health professional is satisfied that the person is fit enough to travel, the opportunities for travel are endless.

Air travel can worsen respiratory problems by causing hypox-aemia. Aircraft cabins are usually pressurised to an altitude of about 2438 m (8000 ft) rather than sea level. At this 'cabin altitude', oxygen blood concentrations in a healthy passenger fall by about 10% to between 7.0 and 8.5 kPa (oxygen saturation 85–91%) but passengers with impaired respiratory function become breathless. The effect is dif-ficult to predict, which may require further investigations before the flight, but guidelines suggest that only patients with severe asthma require an initial assessment. The best predictor of the need for in-flight oxygen is the passenger's oxygen saturation at sea level (i.e. on the ground – see Monitoring Focus, below). Also, people who can walk 50 metres on the level without the need for oxygen, at a steady pace and without feeling breathless or needing to stop, are not likely to be troubled by the reduced pressure in aircraft cabins.

Many insurance companies are reluctant to provide travel insur-ance policies for patients with asthma. A recent poll conducted by Asthma UK found that more than 20% of patients with asthma had been refused insurance, charged an additional premium or had asthma-related events excluded from their policy. Asthma UK can offer advice on travel insurance for people with asthma.

The following advice should be offered to patients with asthma before travelling:

- to carry inhalers in hand luggage and have them at hand at all times
- to take sufficient medicines to last the duration of the holiday plus a few extra days

MONITORING FOCUS

Assessing need for in-flight oxygen[29]	
Oxygen saturation >95%	In-flight oxygen not required
Oxygen saturation 92–95%	
No additional risk factor	In-flight oxygen not required
Hypercapnia, ventilatory support, recent exacerbation, cardiac disease, cerebrovascular disease	Formal assessment of need for in-flight oxygen required
Oxygen saturation <92%	In-flight oxygen required

- to carry with them in their hand language a letter from their doctor that gives details of their conditions and medications
- that a spacer device is as effective as a nebuliser for the delivery of medications (some airlines allow the use of portable nebulisers powered by dry-cell batteries if prior arrangements are made)
- to discuss with their doctor a self-action plan to help recognise symptoms and start treatment (with, for example, prednisolone or antibiotics)
- to take out travel insurance to cover the cost of any unexpected treatments while away.

Sexual health

There is no reason why people with mild-to-moderate asthma should not have a completely normal and healthy sex life. Sex can be a strenuous physical activity, though, and people with asthma should approach it as they would any other form of exercise, taking one or two puffs of their short-acting beta-2 agonist inhaler beforehand.

References

1. Weiss ST, Sparrow D, O'Connor GT. The interrelationship among allergy, airways responsiveness and asthma. *J Asthma* 1993; 30: 329–349.
2. British Thoracic Society/Scottish Intercollegiate Guidelines Network. British Guideline on the Management of Asthma. *Thorax* 2003; 58 (Suppl I): S1–S94.
3. Piacentini GL, Bodini A, Costella A, *et al*. Allergen avoidance is associated with a fall in exhaled nitric oxide in asthmatic children. *J Allergy Clin Immunol* 1999; 104: 1323–1324.
4. Grootendorst DC, Dahlen SE, Va Den Bos JW, *et al*. Benefits of high altitude allergen avoidance in atopic adolescents with moderate to severe asthma, over and above treatment with high dose inhaled steroids. *Clin Exp Allergy* 2001; 31: 400–408.
5. Gotzsche PC, Hammarquist C, Burr M. House dust mite control measures in the management of asthma: meta-analysis. *BMJ* 1998; 317: 1105–1110.
6. Gotzsche PC, Johansen, HK, Hammarquist C, *et al*. House dust mite control measures for asthma (Cochrane Review). *The Cochrane Library*, issue 3. Chichester: John Wiley & Sons, 2001 (*www.thecochranelibrary.com*).
7. Wood RA, Chapman MD, Adkinson NF, *et al*. The effect of cat removal on allergen content in household dust samples. *J Allergy Clin Immunol* 1989; 83: 730–734.
8. Platts-Mills T, Vaughan J, Squillace S, *et al*. Sensitisation, asthma and a modified Th-2 response in children exposed to cat allergen: a population-based cross-sectional study. *Lancet* 2001; 357: 752–756.
9. Althuis MD, Sexton M, Prybylski D. Cigarette smoking and asthma symptom severity among adult asthmatics. *J Asthma* 1999; 36: 257–264.
10. Silvermann RA, Boudreaux ED, Woodruff PG, *et al*. Cigarette smoking among

asthmatics adults presenting to 64 emergency departments. *Chest* 2003; 123: 1472–1479.

11. Siroux V, Pin I, Oryszcyn MP, *et al*. Relationships of active smoking to asthma and asthma severity in the EGEA study. *Eur Respir J* 2000; 15: 470–477.

12. Lange P, Parner J, Vestbo J, *et al*. A 15 year follow-up study of ventilatory function in adults with asthma. *N Engl J Med* 1998; 339; 1194–1200.

13. Chaudhuri R, Livingston E, McMahnon AD, *et al*. Cigarette smoking impairs the therapeutic response to oral corticosteroids in chronic asthma. *Am J Resp Crit Care Med* 2003; 168: 1308–1311.

14. Office of National Statistics 2000. Smoking related attitudes and behaviour, 1999. Series OS no 14.

15. West R, McNeill A, Raw M. Smoking cessation guidelines for health professionals: an update. *Thorax* 2000; 55: 987–999.

16. National Institute for Clinical Excellence. Guidance on the use of nicotine replacement therapy (NRT) and bupropion for smoking cessation. Guidance no. 38, 2002.

17. Committee on the Medical Effects of Air Pollutants. *Asthma and outdoor air pollution*. London: HMSO, 1995.

18. Ernst E. Complimentary therapies for asthma: what patients use. *J Asthma* 1998; 35: 667–671.

19. Stalmatski A. *Freedom from asthma: Buteyko's revolutionary treatment*. London: Kyle Cathie, 1997.

20. Cooper S, Oborne J, Newton S, *et al*. The effect of two breathing exercises (Buteyko and pranayama) in asthma: a randomised controlled trial. *Thorax* 2003; 58: 674–679.

21. Teeter JG, Bleecker ER. Relationship between airway obstruction and respiratory symptoms in adult asthmatics. *Chest* 1998; 113: 277.

22. Carr RE, Leher PM, Rausch LL, *et al*. Anxiety sensitivity and panic attacks in as asthmatic population. *Behav Res Ther* 1994; 32: 411–418.

23. Linde K, Jobst K, Panton J. Acupuncture for chronic asthma (Cochrane Review). *The Cochrane Library*, issue 3. Chichester: John Wiley & Sons, 2001 (*www.thecochranelibrary.com*).

24. Linde K, Jobst KA. Homeopathy for chronic asthma (Cochrane Review). *The Cochrane Library*, issue 3. Chichester: John Wiley & Sons, 2001 (*www.thecochranelibrary.com*).

25. Britton J, Pavord I, Richards K, *et al*. Dietary magnesium, lung function, wheezing and airway hyperreactivity in a random adult population sample. *Lancet* 1994; 344: 357–362.

26. Woods RK, Thien FC, Abramson MJ. Dietary marine fatty acids (fish oil) for asthma (Cochrane Review). *The Cochrane Library*, issue 3. Chichester: John Wiley & Sons, 2001 (*www.thecochranelibrary.com*).

27. Ram FS, Ardern KD. Tartrazine exclusion for allergic asthma (Cochrane Review). *The Cochrane Database of Systematic Reviews* 2001, issue 4. Chichester: John Wiley & Sons, 2001 (www.thecochranelibrary.com).

28. Stenius-Aarniala B, Poussa T, Kvarnstrom J, *et al*. Immediate and long-term effects of weight reduction in obese patients with asthma: randomised controlled study. *BMJ* 2000; 320: 827–832.

29. Stoller JK, Hoisington E, Auger G. A comparative analysis of arranging in flight oxygen abroad commercial air carriers. *Chest* 1999; 115: 991–995.

6

Monitoring asthma

Mortality statistics relating to asthma emphasise the importance of monitoring closely patients' asthma control and their response – or lack of response – to treatment. The severity of asthma can be assessed using relatively simple tests or subjectively by the patient reporting their asthma symptoms. In practice, the patient's symptoms are often recorded and backed up by more objective measurements of lung function, such as peak expiratory flow (PEF).

Symptoms

Symptoms associated with asthma include wheeze, dyspnoea, cough and nocturnal waking. Individual perceptions of each symptom are highly subjective and the health professional relies on accurate patient reporting. Furthermore, several studies have examined the accuracy of patients' perceptions of the severity of their asthma and have highlighted discrepancies between both the patient's and the physician's perception and objective severity. Thus, in those patients who are unable to perceive the severity of their asthma, doctors should check their lung function periodically using an objective measure.

A useful tool to review asthma symptoms collectively is the Royal College of Physicians (RCP) three questions (See Monitoring Focus, page 96).[1] These questions are based on questionnaire responses that correlate with treatment level and are responsive to change. Other tools are available to monitor asthma morbidity such as the Tayside stamp,[2] the Jones morbidity index[3] and Q score.[4]

The Jones morbidity index uses three similar questions to the RCP. It is simple to use and has been shown to be significantly associated with lung function. It is a useful monitoring tool and can be easily used by health professionals, including community pharmacists.[5]

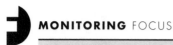

MONITORING FOCUS

Monitoring morbidity: the Royal College of Physicians (RCP) three questions[1] (reproduced with the permission of The RCP)		
In the last week/month	**Yes**	**No**
Have you had difficultly sleeping because of your asthma symptoms (including cough)?		
Have you had your usual asthma symptoms during the day (cough, wheeze, chest tightness, or breathlessness)?		
Has your asthma interfered with your usual activities (e.g. housework, work, school etc.)?		
Date .... / .... /		

- Applies to all patients with asthma aged 16 and over.
- Only use after diagnosis has been established.

Wheeze

A wheeze is a high-pitched audible noise present on either inspiration or expiration. It is produced by air moving at a relatively high speed though an airway that is virtually closed. The walls of the airway flutter, producing the characteristic sound, which can often be heard without a stethoscope. Not all episodes of asthma are accompanied by wheeze. When a wheeze is present, it correlates with airflow obstruction and is significantly associated with lower PEF, although the range of PEF is wide. Thus, wheeze does not lend itself to objective assessment.

Dyspnoea

This symptom is not a sensitive indicator of asthma severity. Airflow obstruction in asthma is greater when the patient exhales air, yet only a small percentage of patients perceive their dyspnoea to be expiratory. Dyspnoea is increased during acute exacerbations and it is thought that the feeling of dyspnoea is related to the effort of breathing rather than to airflow obstruction itself. However, an increase in dyspnoea may indicate to an individual patient that their asthma control is deteriorating.

Cough

Cough is a defence mechanism that protects against aspiration. In human subjects inhalation challenges produce both cough and bronchoconstriction. The two mechanisms appear closely related but are not interdependent. Cough may indicate the presence of asthma but does not necessarily correlate with the severity of airflow obstruction.

Nocturnal waking

The appearance of asthma symptoms during the night and in the early hours of the morning is a sign of worsening asthma. The presence of nocturnal asthma, typically awakening the patient or being present on waking at dawn, correlates strongly with disease activity.

Pulmonary function measurements

Pulmonary function test (PFT) measurements are recommended for the diagnosis of asthma, assessment of severity and to monitor the course of the disease. Although the fully equipped PFT laboratory utilises a host of sophisticated equipment to monitor lung function, simple spirometry and peak flow meters are relatively easy to use and standardise and have become portable enough to use at outreach clinics and in the patient's home.

Peak expiratory flow monitoring

Alyonton and Burge developed the peak flow meter in the 1960s, allowing the measurement of asthma for the first time. Today, the peak flow meter is the most widely used lung function test. It is an extremely simple and cheap test. The peak flow meter records the maximum expiratory flow within the first 2 milliseconds of expiration. The meter is held horizontally and the patient places their lips firmly around the mouthpiece, ensuring that no air escapes. The patient is then asked to take a full inspiration and to then blow out forcefully into the peak flow meter. The best of three tests is recorded (see Monitoring Focus, page 98).

PEF is affected by airway calibre and is effort dependent. The accuracy of this test depends on the individual taking the largest possible intake of breath and making the hardest possible blow out.

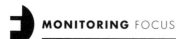

MONITORING FOCUS

Using a peak flow meter

---

1 Connect the mouthpiece to the peak flow meter according to the manufacturer's instructions.
2 Set the marker to the bottom of the numeric scale (closest to the mouthpiece).
3 Stand up if possible, and take as deep a breath as possible.
4 Place lips tightly around the mouthpiece and form a tight seal.
5 Blow out through the mouth as hard and as fast as possible. This will move the main flow indicator up the scale.
6 Note the final position of the marker. This is the peak flow rate.
7 Repeat steps 2–6 twice more, providing three readings altogether.
8 Record the highest peak flow reading of the three.

The peak flow meter is simple to use and can be used by patients at home or work to monitor daily variability in PEF. Repeated measurements throughout the day illustrate the wide diurnal variations in airflow obstruction that characterise asthma (see Figure 6.1).

Home charting of PEF is useful in the following cases:[6]

- at diagnosis and initial assessment
- in assessing response to changes in treatment
- when monitoring response during exacerbations.

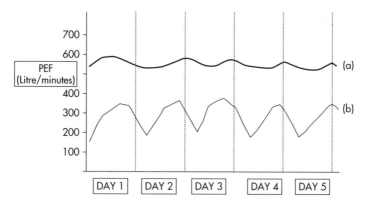

Figure 6.1 Characteristic peak flow chart of a patient with asthma. Peak expiratory flow rate (PEF) shows a circadian rhythm in both normal (a) and asthmatic subjects (b). The variability is greater in an asthmatic subject, PEF typically worsening in the mornings. Increases in diurnal variation are an important indication of poorly controlled asthma.

Not all patients need to monitor their PEF routinely, particularly if their asthma is mild. Patients who would find the measurements useful include those with more severe disease, those with an insidious deterioration of their asthma, those with poor perception of deteriorating dyspnoea and those prone to exacerbations of asthma, who sometimes find PEF useful in taking pre-emptive action. However, in many patients, symptoms alone can be used to detect deterioration, although this will not provide objective measurements of disease severity.

When used in monitoring response to treatments or during exacerbations, the patient's personal best PEF is the most appropriate reference value. To establish the personal best PEF, the peak flow measurement should be taken each day at the same time for 2–3 weeks when the asthma is under control. The patient's personal best PEF may change over time and a new best PEF may need to be established periodically.

Home PEF monitoring should be linked to an appropriate action plan (see Chapter 8). A personalised action plan instructs patients on what action to take if their PEF changes. Such an approach has been shown to lead to better control of asthma.[7]

- Patients who have PEF measurements consistently less than 85% of their best effort may need additional medications to control their asthma.
- A PEF recording of 50–75% of best effort may require the patient to take an oral corticosteroid to gain control of their disease.
- A PEF of less than 50% of best effort indicates a severe exacerbation of asthma and the patient should seek medical help immediately.

In 2004, the Department of Health changed the PEF meters available under the drug tariff to those that meet the new European Union standard (EN 13826).[8] The reliability of these devices is the same as that of the older devices and remains excellent if the device is properly cared for according to the manufacturer's instruction.

In 1991 it was discovered that the original flow calibration was inaccurate, with an over-reading in the middle range of the meters.[9,10] Although PEF that varies throughout the day is characteristic of asthma, the recording of PEF with an inaccurate meter may reduce or enhance the apparent level of variability. One study looked at this effect and confirmed that, in a group of patients with moderate-to-severe asthma, the level of variability and asthma severity was being underestimated in about 30% of patients. By following self-management action plans, these patients were not increasing their treatment appropriately and about 20% more courses of prednisolone would have been started if the PEF values and the assessment of asthma severity had been correct.[11]

The change in meter scale will improve the clinical information derived from these devices, producing accurate PEF measurements across the entire measurement range, similar to those obtained by conventional spirometry. The new meters will give a better assessment of asthma severity for an important number of patients, which should improve asthma care.

Spirometry

Spirometry is a simple method for studying lung function. The spirometer records the volume of air moving in and out of the lungs over time, allowing measurements that relate to the mechanical functioning of the lungs to be calculated (see Figure 6.2 and Monitoring Focus, page 102).

In a sitting position, and wearing a nose clip to prevent air leak, the patient breathes into a mouthpiece connected to the spirometer. To obtain interpretable results from spirometry, it is essential that the

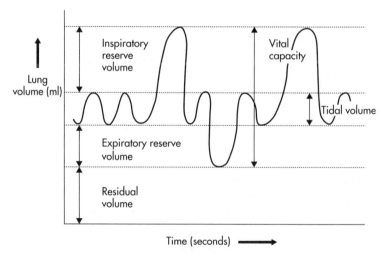

Figure 6.2 Spirometry tracing showing lung volume against time during different breathing conditions. The tidal volume is the volume of air inspired or expired with each normal breath. The inspiratory reserve volume is the amount of air that can be inspired over and above the normal tidal volume; the expiratory reserve volume is the amount of air that can be expelled forcibly after normal tidal expiration. These three values add up to the vital capacity, the maximum amount of air that a person can expel from the lungs after a maximal inspiration.

patient gives full effort during testing. At least three tests of acceptable effort are performed to ensure reproducibility of results; any more than three attempts may exhaust the patient and produce poor results.

Spirometry is a versatile test of pulmonary physiology and is used to measure accurately the degree of airflow obstruction compared with the predicted normal. Accurate measurement of respiratory function is necessary to diagnose, assess and manage asthma appropriately.

Reversibility of airways obstruction can be assessed using a bronchodilator and the spirometer. After spirometry is completed, the patient is given an inhaled bronchodilator and the test is repeated. It can be repeated 5 minutes after administration of the bronchodilator, as a significant improvement in ventilatory function in response to a short-acting beta-2 agonist can be expected within this time. However, most patients require a rest of about 15 minutes after the first measurements.

Before doing a bronchodilatory reversibility test, the patient should be asked to stop their short-acting beta-2 agonist for 6 hours, long-acting bronchodilator for 12 hours and theophyllines for 24 hours.

The purpose of administering a bronchodilator is to assess whether a patient's pulmonary function is responsive to one, by looking for improvement in the expired volumes and flow rates; this can be used to help distinguish between asthma and chronic obstructive airways disease (COPD) where diagnostic doubt remains, or where both COPD and asthma are present.[12] In general, an increase of greater than 15% in the forced expiratory volume in 1 second (FEV_1) (an absolute improvement in FEV_1 of at least 200 mL) or the forced vital capacity (FVC) after inhaling a beta-2 agonist is considered a significant response and is diagnostic of asthma.[6] However, results must be interpreted carefully. The results of a reversibility test performed on different occasions can be inconsistent and not reproducible; over-reliance on a single reversibility test may therefore be misleading unless the change in FEV_1 is greater than 400 mL. The recent COPD management guideline published by the National Institute for Health and Clinical Excellence (NICE)[12] recommends that for a diagnosis of reversible airways disease, the change in FEV_1 following beta-2 agonist inhalation should be greater than 400 mL.

The lack of an acute bronchodilator effect during spirometry does not exclude a response to long-term therapy and further tests may be required.

Spirometry can be used to detect the bronchial hyperreactivity that characterises asthma. By inhaling increasing concentrations of histamine or methacholine, a patient with asthma will demonstrate symptoms and

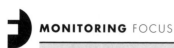

MONITORING FOCUS

Pulmonary function tests – definition of terms

Forced expiratory volume in 1 second (FEV₁)

FEV_1 is the volume of air expelled in the first second of a forced expiration starting from full inspiration. FEV_1 is reduced in obstructive lung disease because of increased airway resistance and in restrictive lung disease because of the low vital capacity.

Forced vital capacity (FVC)

FVC is the total volume of air expelled in the forced expiration starting from full inspiration. Patients with obstructive lung disease usually have a normal or only slightly decreased FVC. Patients with restrictive lung disease (e.g. idiopathic pulmonary fibrosis, kyphoscoliosis and sarcoidosis) have a decreased FVC.

FEV₁/FVC ratio

This is the ratio of the FVC exhaled in the first second of the forced expiration.

- In healthy patients, the FEV_1/FVC ratio is usually above 0.7.
- In patients with obstructive lung disease, the FEV_1/FVC ratio decreases and can be as low as 0.2–0.3 in severe obstructive airway disease.
- FEV_1/FVC ratios are near normal in restrictive airway diseases.

Forced expiratory flow (FEF25–75)

This is the average FEF during the mid (25–75%) portion of the FVC. This is reduced in both obstructive and restrictive airway diseases.

Peak expiratory flow (PEF)

This is the peak flow rate during expiration.

Diffusing capacity of the lung for carbon monoxide (DLCO)

Carbon monoxide can be used to measure the diffusing capacity of the lung, which is decreased in parenchymal lung disease and chronic obstructive airway disease (especially emphysema) but is normal in asthma.

spirometric results consistent with airways obstruction at much lower threshold concentrations than the normal population.

Obtaining useful information from PFTs requires both adequate equipment and reproducible performance. When performing spirometry, it is essential that the patient makes a maximal inspiration and is then instructed and encouraged to blow out as hard as possible and for as long as possible. The most common reason for inconsistent readings is patient technique. Errors may not be apparent by simply looking at values for FEV_1 and FVC but can be detected by observing the patient throughout the manoeuvre and by examining the resultant trace. Common problems include:

- inadequate or incomplete inhalation
- lack of effort during exhalation
- additional breath taken during the manoeuvre
- lips not tight around the mouthpiece
- a slow start to the forced exhalation
- exhalation stops before complete expiration
- some exhalation through the nose
- coughing
- early glottic closure

Flow–volume loops provide a graphic illustration of a patient's spirometric efforts. Flow is plotted against volume to display a continuous loop from inspiration to expiration. The overall shape of the flow–volume loop is important in interpreting spirometric results. The virtually instantaneous peak is the PEF, and the gradually decreasing flow rates follow the progressive airway narrowing down to zero flow rate at a point corresponding to the FVC (the horizontal axis of the flow–volume graph shows the volume expired, equivalent to the FVC). An inspiratory loop can also be obtained by asking the patient to take a maximal intake of breath. The semicircular shape of the normal inspiratory flow curve reflects the time taken for the respiratory muscles to generate maximal inspiratory flow and force. The flow–volume curve can be expressed quantitatively in terms of the flow rate occurring at various volumes. For example, forced expiratory flow values – FEF25 and FEF75 – can be obtained – the average flow (or speed) of air coming out of the lung when 25% and 75% of the FVC volume have been expired. A forced inspiratory flow (FIF) value can be calculated which is similar to the FEF except that the measurement is taken during inspiration.

Figure 6.3 illustrates the four major patterns of flow–volume curve that are obtained.

Obstructive lung diseases such as asthma change the appearance of the flow–volume curve. As with a normal curve, there is a rapid PEF, but the curve descends more quickly than normal and takes on a concave

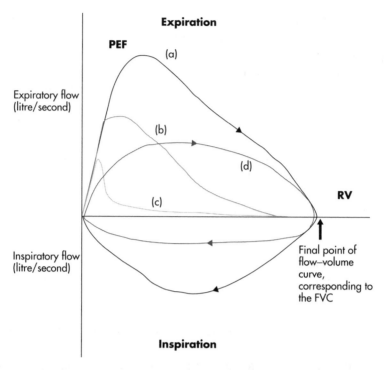

Figure 6.3 Examples of flow–volume loop curves from (a) a healthy adult; (b) a patient with volume-dependent airway narrowing (e.g. asthma); (c) a patient with volume-dependent airway collapse (e.g. chronic obstructive pulmonary disease); (d) a patient with extrathoracic airway obstruction. PEF, peak expiratory flow; RV, residual volume; FVC, forced vital capacity.

shape, reflected by a marked decrease in the FEF25–75. With more severe disease, the peak becomes sharper and the expiratory flow rate drops precipitously. This results from dynamic airway collapse, which occurs as diseased conducting airways are more readily compressed during forced expiratory efforts.

As mentioned above, it is important to examine the curves for operator errors. Variable effort can be detected by a flow–volume loop that fails to demonstrate the normal early peak, showing that the patient did not expire maximally when instructed to do so. Early glottic closure is seen as an abrupt cessation of flow during expiration, visible as a sharp downward slope on the expiratory flow–volume curve. Coughing during spirometry appears as sudden sharp spikes in the decreasing limb of the flow–volume curve.

The volume–time curve is an alternative way to plot spirometric results and is another useful illustration of patient performance. The normal volume–time curve has a rapid upslope and approaches a plateau soon after exhalation. The maximum volume attained represents the FVC, while the volume attained after 1 second represents the FEV_1. The volume–time curve for a patient with an obstructive lung disease such as asthma has a characteristic slower ascent to maximum volume, with a gradual upsloping compared with the rapid rate seen in normal individuals.

Spirometry is typically reported in both absolute values and as a predicted percentage of normal. Normal values vary depending on sex, race, age and height. It is therefore not possible to interpret PFT results without such information. Values for FVC and FEV_1 that are over 80% of predicted are defined as within the normal range. The FEV_1/FVC ratio is expressed as a percentage, and a young individual with normal lung function is able to forcibly expire at least 70% of his/her vital capacity in 1 second (Figure 6.4). A ratio under 70% suggests underlying obstructive physiology. In asthma (an obstructive lung disorder), the FEV_1 is usually decreased, FVC normal and the ratio FEV_1/FVC is decreased (Figure 6.5). In restrictive lung disease, both the FEV_1 and FVC are reduced proportionately and the patient presents with a normal or even elevated FEV_1/FVC ratio (Figure 6.6).

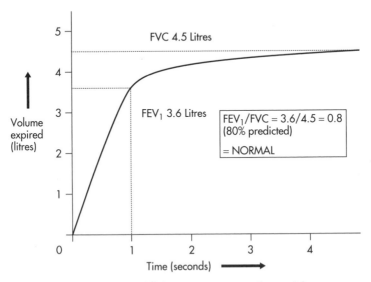

Figure 6.4 Spirometry tracing (volume–time curve) obtained from a patient with normal airways. FVC, forced vital capacity; FEV_1, forced expiratory volume in 1 second.

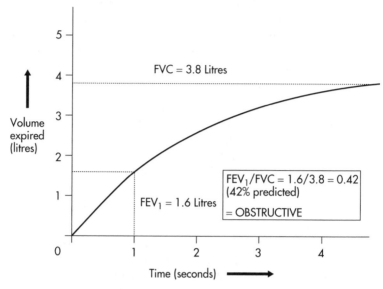

Figure 6.5 Spirometry tracing (volume–time curve) obtained from a patient with asthma or chronic obstructive airway disease – an obstructive picture. FVC, forced vital capacity; FEV$_1$, forced expiratory volume in 1 second.

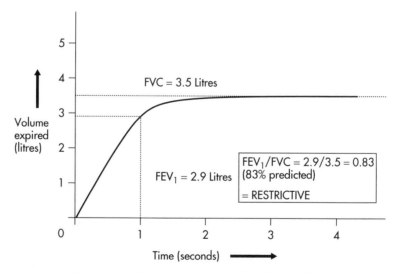

Figure 6.6 Spirometry tracing (volume–time curve) obtained from a patient with idiopathic pulmonary fibrosis – a restrictive picture. FVC, forced vital capacity; FEV$_1$, forced expiratory volume in 1 second.

Spirometry should be performed on initial diagnosis of asthma, after treatment is started and symptoms have stabilised, and every 1–2 years thereafter.

Paediatric lung function testing

Children over 7 years of age can usually perform most PFTs. In children aged 5 years and older, PEF and sometimes FEV_1 and FVC can be measured successfully; however, the child must be encouraged to perform to his/her maximum ability. To help, modern spirometry equipment often has incentive devices that use animated computer software, such as the commercial flow-targeted candle-blowing software, to motivate children to take in as big a breath as possible and blow out as hard as they can. Cooperation in testing is harder to achieve in children under 5 years of age, and alternative means of obtaining information are used. One such technique is the interrupter resistance measurement. This device measures airway resistance to airflow. Higher values suggest reduced calibre (i.e. narrowing of the airways), as seen in conditions such as asthma. The interruption equipment is inexpensive and the test is suitable for 2–5 year olds.[13] The multiple breath washout technique, developed at the Great Ormond Street Hospital, can detect problems in children aged 2–5 years even if they have no respiratory symptoms. The test requires the child to breathe quietly though a facemask for 10–15 minutes. The facemask is connected to a flow meter, which measures the volume of air going into and out of the lungs with each breath.[14] Currently there are no tests to measure lung function accurately in children under 2 years of age.

Pulse oximetry

The measurement of oxygen saturation (SpO_2) by pulse oximetry is necessary in all patients with acute asthma to exclude hypoxaemia.[6] The measurement of SpO_2 enables identification of patients who may be in respiratory failure and therefore in need of more intensive management. The goal of treatment is to maintain SpO_2 above 92%. SpO_2 levels below 92% are an indicator of life-threatening asthma. Supplemental oxygen will be required and detailed blood gas analysis should be performed.

Arterial blood gases

Arterial blood gas measurement provides important information in assessing the severity of asthma exacerbations[6] (see Monitoring focus, page 108). Patients with SpO_2 below 92% or who have other features of life-threatening asthma require measurement of arterial blood gases.

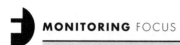

Arterial blood gas measurements

Arterial oxygen tension (PaO_2)

This depends on the ventilation and is affected by the inspired oxygen concentration, ventilatory efficiency and the affinity of blood for oxygen.

- Generally, the more severe the obstruction, the lower PaO_2. A PaO_2 value below 8.0 kPa defines respiratory failure.

Arterial carbon dioxide tension ($PaCO_2$)

- $PaCO_2$ above 6.5 kPa diagnoses hypoventilation.
- $PaCO_2$ below 4.5 kPa diagnosis hyperventilation.

In severe asthma, the patient hyperventilates at first to maintain their PaO_2, causing a reduction in $PaCO_2$. As the patient becomes tired and their breathing slows, the $PaCO_2$ starts to normalise, which should be viewed as a sign of impending respiratory failure. A normal $PaCO_2$ is thus a danger sign in asthma exacerbations.

pH

The pH is a measure of hydrogen ion concentration. The majority of patients with acute asthma have a reduced $PaCO_2$ resulting in a respiratory alkalosis (pH >7.53). As the patient tires, especially in extreme airflow limitation, the $PaCO_2$ increases and metabolic acidosis may result (pH <7.35)

Bicarbonate

Bicarbonate is the most important buffer in the blood. In patients with respiratory alkalosis there may be a slight reduction in plasma bicarbonate concentration (<24 mmol/L), indicating some degree of renal compensation. In severe life-threatening asthma, the raised $PaCO_2$ is compensated by renal retention of bicarbonate ions, returning the pH to within the normal range. This represents a primary respiratory acidosis with a compensatory metabolic alkalosis.

Chest radiograph

A chest radiograph is not routinely recommended but should be performed if any of the following are present:[6]

- suspected pneumomediastinum or pneumothorax
- suspected consolidation
- life-threatening asthma
- failure to respond to treatment satisfactorily
- requirement for ventilation.

Induced sputum

Induction of sputum by inhalation of hypertonic saline has proved to be a reliable and reproducible method of analysing inflammation within the patient's airway. The method of sputum induction is generally safe, although the patient should be monitored for bronchospasm. The collected expectorate is usually examined under a microscope and a differential cell count performed. Induced sputum from normal individuals shows a predominance of macrophages and neutrophils whereas in adults and children with asthma there is an increase in the proportion and number of eosinophils, metachromatic cells and sometimes neutrophils. The degree of eosinophilia increases during asthma exacerbations or through exposure of an atopic patient with asthma to an allergen. Thus, sputum eosinophilia may reflect disease activity, and may prove useful in monitoring asthma severity. In addition, sputum eosinophilia is usually decreased by corticosteroids. Measuring the patient's sputum eosinophils may provide a method to monitor response to and concordance with medication.

Exhaled nitric oxide

Nitric oxide (NO) gas is present in exhaled breath. People with asthma have been shown to have an increased production of NO in their lungs and hence have a higher exhaled NO concentration. Measurement of NO is simple: the patient breathes into a chemiluminescence analyser and the concentration is measured immediately. Levels of NO have been shown to correlate with airway hyperresponsiveness and sputum eosinophil counts, although this was only found in patients not taking corticosteroids. However, elevated NO levels are not specific to asthma and are increased in other respiratory diseases such as bronchiectasis, pulmonary tuberculosis and respiratory tract infections. Measurement of exhaled NO is therefore not recommended to monitor disease severity routinely but could be useful to monitor patient concordance with corticosteroids.

Medication use

The use of symptom-relieving bronchodilators by patients is a good indicator of the severity of their asthma. The asthma management guideline published by the British Thoracic Society and Scottish Intercollegiate Guidelines Network recommends that short-acting beta-2 agonists are prescribed and administered on an as-required basis for shortness of breath, regardless of the severity of asthma.[6] Patients can monitor fluctuations in their bronchodilator use, which may highlight a change in asthma control.

Quality-of-life measures

In a chronic disease such as asthma, health-related quality-of-life (QOL) measures provide an indication of how the disease is affecting the patient[15] and include both physical and psychological assessments of the burden produced by the illness. Specially designed questionnaires (e.g. the Asthma Quality of Life Questionnaire[16]) that are sensitive to changes in asthma control are available for asthma patients. Using this questionnaire, QOL scores have been correlated with morning peak flow[17] and with the severity of asthma.[18] However, in patients with severe asthma, worse-than-expected QOL scores that do not relate with the level of airflow obstruction (as measured by FEV_1 or variation in peak flow) may be obtained.[19] Some improvements in QOL measures are seen with treatment with bronchodilators[20,21] or corticosteroids[22] QOL scores are mainly used in clinical trials but could potentially be useful to measure the overall physical and psychological impact of chronic asthma on the patient, not just the physiological disturbances. Ideally, to obtain a complete picture of a patient's health status, health-related QOL must be measured in conjunction with the conventional clinical measurements – spirometry/PEF measurement and medication requirements, as described above.

References

1. Pearson MG, Bucknall CE, eds. *Measuring Clinical Outcome in Asthma: a Patient-focused Approach*. London: Royal College of Physicians, 1999.
2. Neville RG, Hoskins G, Smith B, *et al.* Observations on the structure, process and clinical outcomes of asthma care in general practice. *Br J Gen Pract* 1996; 46: 583–587.
3. Jones K, Cleary R, Hyland M. Predictive value of a single asthma morbidity index in a general practice population. *Br J Gen Pract* 1999; 49: 23–26.
4. Rimington LD, Davies DH, Lowe D, *et al.* Relationship between anxiety, depression, and morbidity in adult asthma patients. *Thorax* 2001; 56: 266–271.
5. Nishiyama T, Chrystyn H. The Jones Morbidity Index as an aid for community pharmacists to identify poor asthma control during the dispensing process. *Int J Pharm Pract* 2003; 11: 41–46.
6. British Thoracic Society/Scottish Intercollegiate Guidelines Network. British Guideline on the Management of Asthma. *Thorax* 2003; 58 (Suppl I): S1–S94.

7. Lahdensuo A, Haahtela T, Herrala J, *et al.* Randomised comparison of guided self-management and traditional treatment of asthma over one year. *BMJ* 1996; 312: 748–752.

8. Miller MR, Quanjer PhH. Peak flow meters: a problem of scale. *BMJ* 1994; 308: 548–549.

9. Miller MR, Dickinson SA, Hitchings DJ. The accuracy of portable peak flow meters. *Thorax* 1992; 47: 904–909.

10. Gardner RM, Crapo RO, Jackson BR, *et al.* Evaluation of accuracy and reproducibility of peak flow meters at 1400m. *Chest* 1992; 101: 948–952.

11. Miles JF, Tunnicliffe W, Cayton RM, *et al.* Potential effects of correction of inaccuracies of the mini-Wright peak expiratory flow meter on the use of an asthma self-management plan. *Thorax* 1995; 51: 403–406.

12. National Institute for Health and Clinical Excellence (NICE). Chronic obstructive pulmonary disease: national clinical guidance on management of chronic obstructive pulmonary disease in adults in primary and secondary care. *Thorax* 2004; 59 (Suppl 1) : 1–53.

13. Dundas I, McKenzie S. Measurement of lung function in preschool children. *Airways J* 2003; 1: 30–33.

14. Amora P, Bush A, Gustafsson P, *et al.* Multiple breath washout as a marker of lung disease in preschool children with cystic fibrosis. *Am J Respir Crit Care Med* 2005; 171: 249–256.

15. Schrier AC, Dekker FW, Kaptein AA, *et al.* Quality of life in elderly patients with chronic non-specific lung disease seen in family practice. *Chest* 1990; 98: 894–899.

16. Juniper EF, Guyatt GH, Epstein RS, *et al.* Evaluation of impairment of health related quality of life in asthma: development of a questionnaire for use in clinical trials. *Thorax* 1992; 47: 76–83.

17. White EA, Jones PW. Morning and evening peak flow and spirometry as correlates of quality of life in asthma. *Am J Respir Crit Care Med* 1996; 153: A772.

18. Juniper EF, Wiseniewski ME, Cox FM, *et al.* Relationship between quality of life and clinical status is asthma: a factor analysis. *Eur Respir J* 2004; 23: 287–291.

19. Fletcher TJ, Duncanson R, Jones PW, *et al.* Poor quality of life in severe asthma using the AQ20 questionnaire. *Am J Respir Crit Care Med* 1996; 153: A540.

20. Kemp JP, Cook DA, Incaudo GA, *et al.* Salmeterol improves quality of life in patients with asthma requiring inhaled corticosteroids: Salmeterol Quality of Life Study Group. *J Allergy Clin Immunol* 1998; 101(2 pt 1): 188–195.

21. Van der Molen T, Sears MR, de Graaf CS, *et al.* Quality of life during formoterol treatment: comparison between asthma specific and generic questionnaires. Canadian and the Dutch Formoterol Investigators. *Eur Respir J* 1998; 12: 30–34.

22. Juniper EF, Buist SA. Health-related quality of life in moderate asthma: 400 micrograms hydrofluoroalkane beclomethasone dipropionate vs 800 micrograms chlorofluorocarbon beclomethasone dipropionate. *Chest* 1999; 116: 1297–1303.

7

Drug delivery to the lungs

The lungs have a surface area of approximately 100 m^2 and an extensive blood supply, offering an ideal route for drug administration. Inhalation has been used as a method for drug delivery for many years. It was first described in Ayurvedic medicine more than 4000 years ago.[1] The leaves of the plant *Atropa belladonna* (deadly nightshade), which contain atropine, were smoked to treat diseases of the throat and chest. The ancient Greeks and Egyptians supported the use of hot vapours for inhalation purposes and in 1664, Bennett used inhalation therapy for the treatment of tuberculosis. During the 1800s, vapours released from various aromatic plants, balsams and sulfur were used for the treatment of chest infections, and later that century Potter's asthma cigarettes became popular. These contained tobacco mixed with shredded leaves from the plant *Datura stramonium* (a poisonous tropical weed, commonly known as thorn apple) which caused a bronchodilator effect analogous to that seen with the inhalation of ipratropium bromide by aerosol.

The nebuliser was developed in the late 1820s as an inhalation device for liquid droplets. The inhalation of nebulised aerosols was advertised as beneficial for many conditions, such as pharyngitis, laryngitis, bronchitis, pain, catarrh, asthma, tuberculosis and sleeplessness. The liquids and substances inhaled varied widely and included mineral water containing sulfur, iodine and chlorine; sedatives; antiseptics; and belladonna. The development and use of adrenaline (epinephrine) in the treatment of asthma was a major advance. In 1911, adrenaline was mixed with water and glycerol and given via nebuliser to treat respiratory conditions. However, the adverse effects from adrenaline curtailed its use and it was replaced in clinical practice in 1951 by isoprenaline.

The most important development in delivery of anti-asthma drugs was the advent of the metered-dose inhaler (MDI) in 1956, which resulted in a huge increase in the use of anti-asthma therapies. Since then the technology of inhaled drug delivery has advanced to include dry-powder inhalers (DPIs). However, further developments of devices with better delivery to the lungs are still needed. Sales of MDIs now run at approximately 500 million units per year and the worldwide market for inhaled therapy is expected to reach £5 billion by 2008.[3]

The major advantage of topical administration of a drug is the possibility of achieving a high local concentration whilst avoiding high systemic concentrations. To deposit a drug in the airways, it must be aerolised, which is achieved by the inhalation system. MDIs, DPIs and nebulisers are the currently used delivery systems. Health professionals involved in prescribing aerosol therapy must be well informed about these systems in order to make appropriate choices for their patients.

Factors that affect the clinical outcome from aerosol therapy

The amount of topically available drug is determined by a number of factors:

- the delivery characteristics of the inhaler
- handling of the device
- inhalation technique of the patient
- patient preference for a particular inhaler
- concordance with the inhaler.

Successfully delivery of drugs to the lungs presents one of the most challenging design tasks in pharmaceutical formulation.

Factors affecting drug deposition

For a drug that is inhaled as an aerosol to exert its effect, drug particles must be deposited in the lungs. MDIs are relatively inefficient since typically only 10–20% of the actuated drug is deposited in the lungs; 70–80% is swallowed and up to 10% exhaled. Factors affecting deposition in the airways include:

- the size of the particles that come out of the device
- the inspiratory flow rate
- the patient's inhalational technique
- use of inhaler attachments (e.g. spacers).

These variables are discussed below.

Particle size

The following are the approximate diameters of sections of the respiratory tract:

- trachea, 1.8 cm
- bronchioles, 0.5 cm
- terminal bronchioles and alveoli, 0.04–0.06 cm.

The particle size of the aerosol is an important factor affecting deposition in the lungs, both in terms of quantity of the drug deposited and the site of drug deposition. Particle size is conventionally described in terms of the mass median aerodynamic diameter (MMD) – the value exceeded by 50% of particles. Particles of greater than 10 micrometres are likely to be deposited in the oropharynx; those of 5–10 micrometres reach the larger airways and those of 2–5 micrometres reach the small airways. Particles of 0.5–2 micrometres are deposited in the alveoli, while those less than 0.5 micrometres in diameter are exhaled. Particles of 2–5 micrometres are ideal for drug delivery. At this MMD, fewer particles are swallowed and lung deposition is more even.[3–5]

Differences in pulmonary deposition between devices have been reported even when an optimal inhalation technique is used, varying from approximately 5% for the Spinhaler, 7–20% for MDIs, 20–30% for the Turbohaler and 38% for MDIs used in combination with large-volume spacers.[6–8]

Depending on the drug and device used, some of the drug will impact on the tongue or back of the pharynx. This portion will be swallowed (unless the patient rinses his or her mouth) and may be absorbed from the gastrointestinal tract, although some may be inactivated by first-pass metabolism in the liver. Only the fraction escaping this reaches the systemic circulation, where it has the capacity to produce side-effects. The percentage of drug deposited in the lung from the device is therefore an important consideration when reviewing the potential side-effects of an inhaled drug. However, a proportion of drug will also be absorbed via the lungs and adds to the systemic effects of the drug.

Accurate measurement of the particle size of an aerolised drug from *in vitro* studies may help predict the *in vivo* behaviour and clinical effect of the drug. However, many other factors influence pulmonary deposition, such as the inertia of the particles, sedimentation or settling, and the effects of solvents and propellants. Patient-related factors will also affect particle deposition, such as respiratory tract anatomy and changes in breathing patterns. Therefore, determination of the therapeutic equivalence of different formulations should not rely on *in vitro* measurements alone.

Difference in drug delivery can also make it difficult to interpret data from clinical trials. Trials should not be grouped in a meta-analysis without considering differences in the delivery devices.

Inspiratory flow rate

Inspiratory flow rate is also an important variable: higher flow rates increase central airways deposition while a slower rate of inspiration and breath-holding increases peripheral deposition.

Assessment of inspiratory flow provides an opportunity to educate and review inhaler use; determining whether a patient can obtain the optimum inspiratory flow rate for a device can be a significant step towards optimising treatment. For some patients, it reveals their inability to use a particular device, alerting health professionals to a likely reason for poor response to treatment.

Patients who cannot achieve the optimum inspiratory flow for their inhaler may not gain maximum benefit from prescribed medication, and health professionals may wish to take this factor into account when selecting a particular type of inhaler. For example, pulmonary deposition decreases by 50% if the flow used to inhale from a Turbohaler device is reduced from a normal flow of 60 litres/minute to a suboptimal flow of 30 litres/minute.[8]

Recognition of sub-optimal inhalation is more difficult than many realise, and experienced respiratory professionals now accept that without an objective test, a visual observation of technique is no more accurate than a guess. Many inspiratory flow meters are available that can be used to calculate a person's inspiratory flow.

For each type of inhaler, the most effective delivery – and thus the most desirable or most beneficial outcome for the patient – occurs when the patient achieves a flow within the optimum inspiratory flow range (see Inhalation Delivery Focus, page 117).

Inhalational technique

The patient's inhalation technique is likely to be the single most important factor in determining the efficacy of treatment. Use of a manually actuated MDI requires good coordination and psychomotor skills to ensure that actuation, inhalation and breath-holding occur in precise sequence. Studies have shown that some 75% of patients do not use their MDI correctly.[17] Common errors: are not shaking the canister

INHALATIONAL DELIVERY FOCUS

Optimum inspiratory flow rates for inhaler devices[8-16]	
Inhaler device	**Optimum inspiratory flow rate (litres/minute)**
Turbohaler	60–90
Accuhaler	30–90
Clickhaler	15–60
Easibreathe	20–60
Autohaler	30–60
Metered-dose inhaler	25–60

before use, inhaling too rapidly, and not holding the breath for long enough at the end of inspiration. A further problem is the 'cold Freon' effect, where the impact of the cold propellant on the back of the throat may cause the patient to halt inspiration and induce coughing. As a result, insufficient drug reaches the airways, impairing effectiveness and increasing the risk of local adverse effects.

The mechanisms of particle deposition dictate how an inhaler device should be used. Breathing the aerosol in slowly and deeply reduces the amount of impaction in the mouth and pharynx and allows the particles to travel into the smaller airways. The patient holds their breath after slowly inhaling the aerosol to give the particles time to deposit by sedimentation and diffusion. If the breath is not held, the very small particles (MMD <1 micrometre) that rely on deposition by diffusion, along with a proportion of the slightly larger ones (MMD approximately 5 micrometres) that have not had time to settle, will be exhaled.

Inhaler attachments

There are two types of attachments for inhalers: the extension device and the holding chamber (spacer devices), the latter being the most commonly used. These attachments provide a reservoir of drug from which the patient breathes. This increases the deposition of the drug in the lower airways by allowing evaporation of propellant, thereby creating more droplets of a respirable size. They also reduce oro-pharyngeal deposition by allowing large particles to impact within the device. This is particularly useful for inhaled corticosteroids where there is potential for local adverse effects. Finally, by acting as a holding chamber for the aerosol, these devices allow the patient to inhale the drug over several breaths, making coordination less critical. They are generally easier for children and older, frailer patients to use than a conventional MDI alone. Facemasks with holding chambers are particularly helpful for very young children with asthma although drug delivery is more efficient via a mouthpiece if the patient can use one.[8]

To administer a drug, a single actuation into the spacer should be inhaled with minimum delay after each puff, repeating until the prescribed dose has been taken. The canister should be shaken between doses. Either a single slow, deep inspiration or a series of smaller breaths, known as tidal breathing, can be used and have been shown to be equally effective.[8]

Static charge will accumulate on the walls of any holding chamber made of plastic. This attracts drug particles and reduces the output of the medication from the chamber, reducing the efficacy of the drug. Washing the spacer in washing-up liquid, and allowing it to dry naturally in air without wiping reduces the static charge and increases the delivery of the drug to the lungs.[19] The use and care of holding chambers (spacers) is summarised in the Inhalation Delivery Focus below.

Patient preference

The development of new devices has generated a number of studies looking at patient preference for a particular inhaler. Although it is

INHALATIONAL DELIVERY FOCUS

Use and care of holding chambers (spacers) with metered-dose inhalers (MDIs)[20]

- The spacer should be compatible with the MDI being used.
- The drug should be administered by repeated single actuations of the MDI into the spacer, each followed by inhalation.
- There should be minimal delay between actuation and inhalation.
- Tidal breathing is as effective as single breaths.
- Spacers should be cleaned monthly rather than weekly according to the manufacturer's recommendations, otherwise performance is adversely affected.
- Spacers should be washed in detergent and allowed to dry in air. The mouthpiece should be wiped clean of detergent before use.
- Drug delivery may vary significantly because of static charge. Metal and other antistatic spacers have been shown to be effective in reducing static charge.
- Spacers should be replaced at least every 12 months but some may need changing earlier than this if a white film appears on the inside of the spacer and/or around the mouthpiece.

reasonable to suggest that preference for one or another device may affect patient concordance, this has not been clinically shown. It should be borne in mind that studies looking at a particular device are often sponsored by the manufacturer, and the questionnaire used tends to be biased in favour of their own products.

Patient concordance

Poor concordance can have a detrimental effect on the patient's control of their asthma. It is a major cause of apparent treatment failure and results in excess mortality. Clinically studies in which inhalers equipped with electronic monitoring systems were used have indicated that up to 40% of patients tend to under-use and about 20% over-use their medication, despite adequate supervision. It has been shown that concordance can be improved by regular instruction and education, as well as reducing the number of daily inhalations.[21,22]

Handling and maintenance of the inhaler

The way in which the patient handles the device should be taught and practised, and checked regularly, as incorrect handling affects the efficacy of the treatment. For example, laboratory-based studies have shown that neglecting to shake the MDI before use reduces the total particle dose by 25%, while two actuations 1 second apart decreased fine particle dose by 16%.[18] The same authors also demonstrated that storing the MDI with the stem downwards reduced the total particle dose of the next actuation by 23%. Storing an inhaler in a humid environment also decreases the fine particle fraction, which may affect the clinical outcome. This has been demonstrated with the Turbohaler and Accuhaler devices. Furthermore, it has been shown that the increase in forced expiratory flow in 1 second was 80% of maximum achievable after inhalation from the unprimed MDI, compared with 92% after inhalation from the primed one.[23]

Inhaler devices

Inhaler devices can be divided into three groups; different devices suit different patients:

- MDIs
- DPIs
- nebulisers

Metered-dose inhalers

MDIs contain the drug dissolved or suspended in a propellant under pressure. Following actuation, a metered volume of drug and propellant is released, the propellant providing the force to propel and disaggregate particles. As the droplets move away from the release valve, the propellant evaporates, leaving drug particles suspended in air. Unfortunately, however, evaporation is not instantaneous, and because of the speed with which the aerosol is released, the majority of the dose is deposited in the oropharynx before the propellant evaporates completely. Traditionally, the propellants used in the MDI have been chlorofluorocarbons (CFCs) but these are gradually being replaced by ozone-friendly propellants such as hydrofluoroalkanes (HFAs).

MDIs can be manually actuated or breath actuated. Manual MDIs (see Figure 7.1) have been available since the late 1950s and are still by far the most commonly used inhaler device. In 1998, about 80% of inhalers dispensed on prescription in England were MDIs. MDIs are inexpensive compared with other devices, are easily portable and do not require reloading between doses. They can be used alone or in combination with various adaptators (e.g. holding chambers, spacer devices). The advantages and disadvantages of MDIs are summarised in the Inhalation Delivery Focus on page 121.

Breath-actuated MDIs (see Figure 7.2), for example Autohaler and Easi-Breathe, incorporate a mechanism that releases the drug when the patient inhales through the mouthpiece. Such devices can be activated at relatively low inspiratory flow rates of about 30 litres/minute, making

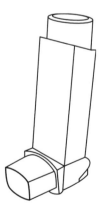

Figure 7.1 A manually actuated metered-dose inhaler.

INHALATIONAL DELIVERY FOCUS

Advantages and disadvantages of metered-dose inhalers (MDIs)	
Advantages	**Disadvantages**
• Small and portable • Usually cheap • Rapid to use • Multi-dose	• Good coordination is essential. • Children under 6 years of age cannot use them without a holding chamber. • Elderly patients and those with arthritis or with coordination problems may not be able to use them without additional aids. A device like the Haleraid may be useful. The Haleraid fits onto some MDIs and allows medicine to be released by applying pressure with the palm of the hand, which can be easier than pressing the canister down. • Few MDIs have a dose counter, making it difficult to know when a new prescription is needed.

them more effective for elderly patients and those experiencing an acute asthma attack, and they do not require coordination of actuation and inspiration. In one study, lung deposition of salbutamol was significantly greater in patients using a breath-actuated MDI than in patients using a manually actuated MDI with poor technique.[15] In those with good technique, however, the breath-actuated MDI offers no advantage.

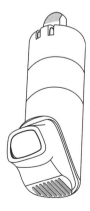

Figure 7.2 A breath-actuated metered-dose inhaler.

Switch to chlorofluorocarbon-free devices

Traditionally, MDIs have contained CFC propellants. However, CFCs are the subject of an international agreement, the Montreal Protocol, which aims to phase out production of these chemicals because of their association with depletion of stratospheric ozone, prompting the development of alternative propellants – HFAs – that are much less damaging to the ozone layer. The first CFC-free MDI, Airomir salbutamol, was introduced in 1995, followed by other CFC-free salbutamol MDIs such as Salbulin, Airomir autohaler and Ventolin Evohaler. With regard to the inhaled corticosteroids, fluticasone is manufactured as a CFC-free preparation but only one CFC-free beclometsaone MDI inhaler is currently available – QVAR –, licensed as a manually or breath-actuated MDI for use in patients aged 12 years and over. The new inhalers are used in just the same way as CFC-containing MDIs. However, patients may notice that HFA inhalers feel or taste different to their CFC counterparts, and devices may also sound different on actuation.

CFC formulations will still be prescribable until a choice of CFC-free alternatives is available for all patient groups at an adequate range of doses, and devices have undergone a year's post-marketing surveillance. It is essential that the changeover is managed carefully and is accompanied by education schemes so that patients understand the reason for the change. Good communication between hospital doctors, general practitioners, practice nurses, pharmacists and patients during the transition is essential.

Dry-powder inhalers

In DPIs the drug is formulated as a dry powder without a propellant. Inspiratory airflow releases the powder and disperses the drug into small particles and delivers it to the lungs. There is no need for coordination between inspiration and actuation of the device. The devices differ in how inspiratory flow affects particle size and delivery to the lungs. Patients should be monitored carefully in terms of symptom control and systemic adverse effects if switching from one type of DPI to another. Oropharyngeal deposition is usually high and patients should be advised to rinse the mouth and throat with water after inhaling from a DPI in order to reduce local side-effects and absorption. The advantages and disadvantages of DPIs are summarised in the Inhalational Delivery Focus on page 124. The DPI devices licensed for use in the UK are listed in the Inhalational Delivery Focus on page 124 and examples of such devices are illustrated in Figure 7.3.

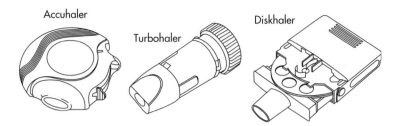

Figure 7.3 Examples of dry-powder inhalers.

Diskhaler and Accuhaler

The Diskhaler and Accuhaler are multidose inhaler devices. They have been designed to deliver a similar dose to that received from a correctly used MDI without a spacer attachment. Both inhalers contain lactose (or glucose) which acts as a carrier. This has a distinctive taste and the patient is reassured that the dose has been taken.

Turbohaler

The Turbohaler is a multidose inhaler device that delivers the pure drug with no carrier admixture. The drug is tasteless, however, which some patients find disconcerting because they worry that they have not received the dose. Patients should be told to inhale forcefully and deeply. With a good inspiratory flow rate (approximately 60 litres/minute), lung deposition is twice that achieved with the same dose inhaled correctly from an MDI. The dose reaching the lungs decreases by 50% when the inspiratory flow rate falls to 30–40 litres/minute, which is still comparable with that achieved with a MDI. A desiccant is stored in the base of the Turbohaler to ensure that the interior of the device and dry powder remain dry. When the inhaler is not being used, the watertight cover must be screwed back in place to protect the inhaler against moisture.

Prescribing devices

Selection of the most appropriate device for a patient is an important decision (see Inhalation Delivery Focus, page 125). Incorrect use (or no use) of an inhaler is a common reason for treatment failure. In the UK, the majority of patients should be initially prescribed an MDI, with a holding chamber recommended for high-dose inhaled corticosteroids and for any patient who has difficulty with coordination. There is no

INHALATIONAL DELIVERY FOCUS

Advantages and disadvantages of dry-powder inhalers	
Advantages	**Disadvantages**
• Small and portable • Coordination between priming and inspiration is not important • Can be used by children without the need for a bulky holding chamber • Multidose	• Lung deposition depends on inspiratory flow • Generally more expensive than metered-dose inhalers

INHALATIONAL DELIVERY FOCUS

Dry-powder devices licensed in the UK	
Dry-powder inhaler	**Generic drug available (brand name)**
Diskhaler	Salbutamol (Ventodisks) Salmeterol (Serevent) Beclometasone (Becodisks) Fluticasone (Flixotide)
Pulvinal	Salbutamol Beclometasone
Cyclohaler	Salbutamol Beclometasone
Clickhaler	Salbutamol (Asmasal) Beclometasone (Asmabec)
Turbohaler	Terbutaline (Bricanyl) Formoterol (Oxis) Budesonide (Pulmicort) Formoterol with budesonide (Symbicort)
Twisthaler	Mometasone (Asmanex)
Accuhaler	Salbutamol (Ventolin) Salmeterol (Serevent) Fluticasone (Flixotide) Salmeterol with Fluticasone (Seretide)
Handihaler	Tiotropium (Spiriva)
Aerocaps	Ipratropium (Atrovent)
Spinhaler	Sodium cromoglicate (Intal)

evidence to support a particular order in which devices should be tried for those patients who cannot use an MDI. The asthma management guideline developed by the British Thoracic Society and Scottish Intercollegiate Guidelines Network (BTS/SIGN) recommends the following when prescribing an inhaler device (bearing in mind that the choice of device may be determined by the choice of drug).[20]

- If the patient is unable to use a device satisfactorily, an alternative should be found.
- The patient's ability to use an inhaler should be assessed by a competent health professional.
- The medication needs to be titrated against clinical response to ensure optimum efficacy.
- The patient's inhalational technique should be reassessed as part of structured clinical review.

 INHALATIONAL DELIVERY FOCUS

Age-specific recommendations for prescribing of inhaler devices[8,20]			
Age (years)	First choice	Second choice	Comments
0–2	MDI plus spacer and facemask	Nebuliser	Ensure optimum spacer used
3–<5	MDI plus spacer	Nebuliser	A facemask is required until the child can breathe reproducibly using the spacer mouthpiece
5–12	MDI plus spacer	Breath-actuated MDI or DPI	MDI plus spacer is as effective as any other hand-held inhaler device If patient prefers DPI or breath-actuated MDI, also consider MDI plus spacer for acute exacerbations
over 12	MDI plus spacer	Breath-actuated MDI or DPI	Spacer device recommended, especially for high-dose inhaled corticosteroids

MDI, metered-dose inhaler; DPI, dry-powder inhaler.

Nebulisers

A nebuliser converts drug solution into a continuous fine aerosol mist of droplets, normally 1–5 micrometres in diameter, which can be inhaled directly into the lungs via a mouthpiece or facemask. The nebuliser is a small plastic device that contains the drug solution and is driven by a compressor (electric or battery operated) or a supply of compressed air or oxygen. A flow of gas of 6–8 litres/minute is normally required to drive the nebuliser. Drug inhalation is accomplished by normal tidal breathing over a 10–15 minute period and not, as with hand-held devices, by deep and usually rapid inhalation.

Indications for use of nebuliser treatment in asthma have declined (see Inhalational Delivery Focus, below).[24] However, nebulisers do offer some advantages: they do not rely on patient cooperation or coordination, allowing patients who are too ill, short of breath or otherwise unable to use a hand-held inhaler to self-administer drug therapy. Nebulisers can be useful when large doses of drug are needed or when drugs intended for the lungs are not available in hand-held inhalers (e.g. antibiotics for patients with cystic fibrosis).

Although nebulisers are easy to use, they are inefficient in drug delivery. In practice, nebulisers vary greatly in the amount of drug delivered in the respirable range, and with many nebulisers less than 10% of the prescribed dose reaches the lungs. Particles larger than 5 micrometres will deposit in the nasopharynx and those smaller than 1 micrometres are likely to be exhaled without impacting in the smaller airways. There is little data on drug deposition from different systems, particularly in children.

INHALATIONAL DELIVERY FOCUS

Indications for nebulised therapy in asthma[26]

- Treatment of severe acute asthma with beta-2 agonist and anticholinergic in hospital
- Supervised treatment of acute severe asthma in the home by a general practitioner
- Treatment of acute severe asthma in an ambulance
- Domiciliary treatment of acute asthma in young children
- Reserve emergency treatment for selected adults with refractory ('brittle') asthma

---

Some patients have nebulisers at home and this may occasionally be appropriate. The danger is that patients rely on their nebuliser to give bronchodilators when symptoms are severe enough to warrant corticosteroids. It is thus essential that patients understand the limitations of the device. Acute attacks of asthma can be treated as effectively with multiple doses of bronchodilator given by MDI and a holding chamber.

Nebulisers and compressors are not available on NHS prescription. Respiratory experts recommend that patients are discouraged from buying their own equipment and should be referred to a clinician to access appropriateness. Many respiratory centres can provide nebuliser units and service them without charge if the nebuliser is deemed essential to the patient's therapy.

The two main types of nebuliser are the jet nebuliser and the ultrasonic nebuliser.

Jet nebulisers

Jet nebulisers are the most common type used in hospitals, general practice and in patients' homes. The flow of gas through a narrow opening (or venturi) creates a negative pressure that draws up drug solution from a reservoir, forming a mist for the patient to inhale. Larger particles deposit on the side of the nebuliser chamber and fall back into the reservoir to be recycled.

A major factor affecting droplet size is the flow rate of gas to the nebuliser. Generally, flow rates below 6 litres/minute will not produce an adequate distribution of respirable particles. If using cylinder oxygen to drive a nebuliser, for example for an acute asthma attack, a regulator designed to produce a flow rate over 6 litres/minute should be used (standard oxygen cylinders have flow rates of either 2 or 4 litres/minute). Other factors that affect drug deposition from a nebuliser include the duration of nebulisation, the nature of the solution or suspension being nebulised and the amount of liquid in the chamber of the nebuliser. For clinical purposes, it is essential to be aware of the driving gas flow rate at which the nebuliser functions most efficiently.

When using a standard jet nebuliser, over half the dose is lost during exhalation. Advanced jet nebulisers (produced by Medic-Aid [Sidestream, Ventstream] and Pari [Pari LC Plus]) improve the efficiency of drug delivery to the lungs. The Sidestream enhances the amount of drug nebulised: an inlet vent draws air into the nebuliser, which increases the rate of flow of nebulised drug, allowing lower specification compressors (with lower flow rates) to be used with this device. The Ventstream and Pari LC Plus nebulisers reduce wastage of drug; these nebulisers are breath assisted, which means that aerosol production is boosted during inspiration and reduced during expiration. These nebulisers are suitable for more viscous drug solutions such as corticosteroids and antibiotics.

One of the most recent developments in nebuliser technology is a system known as the adaptive aerosol delivery system, the HaloLite, which delivers a precise dose and then switches itself off. This device adapts to the patient's individual breathing pattern and delivers during inspiration only, thereby reducing wastage of drug.

Ultrasonic nebulisers

In these nebulisers a rapidly vibrating piezo crystal in the reservoir forms a fountain of liquid from which the aerosol mist arises. The particle size of the generated aerosol varies depending on the frequency of the ultrasonic vibrations. In general, ultrasonic nebulisers are less efficient for drug delivery than jet nebulisers. These nebulisers do not nebulise drug suspensions efficiently.

Issues to consider with nebuliser use

Nebulisation time
The nebulisation time is the time from starting nebulisation until continuous nebulisation has ceased. The time taken to deliver a drug is important for concordance. Nebulisation time for bronchodilators should be less than 10 minutes.

The nebulisation end point is difficult for patients to recognise. Patients need to know how long drug delivery should take when their equipment is working correctly and should be advised to nebulise for about a minute after 'spluttering' occurs. Tapping the nebuliser chamber when the solution begins to splutter will increase the volume output.

Fill and residual volumes
The fill volume is the total amount of solution put into the nebuliser chamber; the residual volume is the amount of liquid remaining in the nebuliser chamber when nebulisation has ceased. If 2 ml of drug solution is nebulised fully from a nebuliser with a residual volume of 1 ml, a maximum of 50% of the drug will be released as aerosol (as 1 ml of the drug solution remains in the chamber). If 4 ml of drug solution is placed in the chamber, a maximum of 75% can be released.

These volumes vary with different nebuliser systems. If the residual volume is less than 1 ml, a fill volume of 2.0–2.5 ml may be adequate. Nebulisers with residual volumes of more than 1 ml generally require fill volumes of about 4 ml. If the drug has to be diluted before nebulisation to achieve the fill volume recommended for the particular nebuliser, normal saline (i.e. 0.9%) should be used to maintain isotonicity. Hypertonic solutions have been reported to produce bronchospasm. The volume of drug solution must not exceed the maximum fill volume. The larger the fill volume, the longer the nebulisation time.

Mouthpiece or facemask?
A mouthpiece is the preferred method for delivery of nebulised drugs to the lungs, which can increase aerosol by up to 85%. Facemasks allow more contact of drug with the skin of the face, possibly causing allergic reactions. However, masks are likely to be the only means of delivering nebulised drugs to infants. The child's face should be washed after delivery of nebulised steroids via a facemask. Nebulised ipratropium bromide, via a facemask, may result in an adverse affect on intra-ocular pressure, potentially leading to acute-angle-closure glaucoma.

Cleaning
At home, nebulisers and the mouthpiece or facemask should be washed in warm soapy water after each use. Tubing should be kept dry. Before commencing a new dose, the nebuliser should be allowed to run for 10 seconds to remove any residual fluid. Equipment should always be maintained according to the manufacturer's recommendations.

Hospital departments need to maintain a reliable nebuliser loan service and provide patients with information, an agreement to service equipment and an emergency loan facility in case equipment fails.

Future developments in pulmonary delivery

The market for inhaler devices may seem overcrowded, but many companies are exploring the development of more effective devices. Many new types of DPI and MDI are under development, some offering very precise drug delivery to the airways via electronic systems. However, devices are likely to be expensive and they are therefore unlikely to replace the cheaper traditional devices.

A novel inhaler developed by Boehringer Ingelheim is the Respimat soft-mist inhaler, a delivery device for the combination of fenoterol and ipratropium bromide. Respimat is a propellant-free, liquid-based device that produces a slow-moving mist of drug. The soft mist travels more slowly and lasts much longer than aerosol clouds from traditional devices, and scintigraphic studies show that this leads to greater drug deposition in the lungs and less in the mouth and throat than with an MDI. A review of clinical trials suggests that it may be possible to reduce the dose of ipratropium/fenoterol required for the same efficacy than when treatment is inhaled through a CFC-based MDI.[25]

SkyeHaler, a DPI developed by drug-delivery specialists SkyePharma, has received approval in the European Union for use with formoterol. It uses magnesium stearate to protect dry-powder drugs from moisture and, in the case of formoterol, to help bulk up the low doses that are required, so that flow and deposition can be improved.

The Nektar pulmonary inhaler is powered by a bolus of compressed air to make drug delivery independent of inspiratory air flow, and the powder is dispersed into a holding chamber from which the patient inhales.[26] Like many of the new generation of inhalers, the Nektar device includes an indicator to show when a dose has been taken.

Another novel approach aimed at improving the delivery of drug to the lung is the SmartMist, a microprocessor-controlled device that enables actuation of an MDI at a pre-programmed point during inspiration, with a traffic-light system to signal when the patient has inhaled correctly. It also measures lung function, with a downloadable record of results.[27,28]

Vectura has developed the Gyrohaler, which is smaller, lighter and easier to use than any other DPI and has the added advantage of being inexpensive.

References

1. Gandevia B. Historical review of the use of parasympathicoltyic agents in the treatment of respiratory disorders. *Postgrad Med J* 1975; 51: 13–20.
2. Muthu DC. *Pulmonary Tuberculosis: Its Etiology and Treatment – Record of twenty-two years observation and work in open-air sanatoria*. London: Baillière, Tindall and Cox, 1922.
3. Bisgaard H, O'Callaghan C, Smaldone GC, eds. *Drug Delivery to the Lung*. Marcel Dekker Inc., New York 2002.
4. Matthys H. Inhalation delivery of asthma drugs. *Lung* 1990 (Suppl): 168: 645–652.
5. Pederen S. Inhalers and nebulisers: which to choose and why. *Respir Med* 1996; 90: 69–77.
6. Pauwels R, Newman S, Borgstrom L. Airway deposition and airway effects of antiasthma drugs delivered from metered dose inhalers. *Eur Respir J* 1997; 10: 2127–2138.

7. Thorsson L, Kenyon C, Newman S, *et al*. Lung deposition of budesonide in asthmatics: a comparison of different formulations. *Int J Pharm* 1998; 158: S146–S153.

8. Inhaler devices for asthma. *Drug Ther Bull* 2000; 38(2): 9–14.

9. Newman S, Moren F, Trofast E, *et al*. Terbutaline sulphate Turbohaler: effect of inhaled flow rate on drug deposition and efficacy. *Int J Pharm* 1991; 74: 209–213.

10. Hill LS, Slater AL. A comparison of the performance of two modern multidose dry powder asthma inhalers. *Resp Med* 1998; 92: 105–110.

11. Nielson K G, Auk I L, Bojsen K, *et al*. Clinical effect of Diskus dry-powder inhaler at low and high inspiratory flow rates in asthmatic children. *Eur Resp J* 1998; 11: 350–354.

12. Malton A, Sumby BS, Dandiker Y. A comparison of in-vitro drug delivery from salbutamol Diskus and terbutaline Turbohaler inhalers. *J Pharm Med* 1996; 6: 35–48.

13. Engel T, Heinig JH, Madsen F, *et al*. Peak inspiratory flow and inspiratory vital capacity of patients with asthma measured with and without a new dry-powder inhaler device (Turbohaler). *Eur Resp J* 1990; 3: 1037–1041.

14. Newhouse MT, Nantel NP, Chambers CB, *et al*. Clickhaler (a novel dry powder inhaler) provides similar bronchodilation to pressurised metered-dose inhaler, even at low flow rates. *Chest* 1999; 115: 952–956.

15. Newman SP, Weisz AWB, Talaee N, *et al*. Improvement of drug delivery with a breath actuated pressurised aerosol for patients with poor inhaler technique. *Thorax* 1991; 46: 712–716.

16. Ross DL, Schultz RK. Effect of inhalation flow rate on the dosing characteristics of dry powder inhaler (DPI) and metered dose inhaler (MDI) products. *J Aerosol Med* 1996; 9(2): 215–226.

17. Goodman DE. The influence of age, diagnosis and gender on proper use of metered dose inhalers. *Am J Resp Crit Care Med* 1994; 150: 1256–1261.

18. Everard ML, Devadason SG, Summers QA, *et al*. Factors affecting total and "respirable" dose delivered by a salbutamol metered dose inhaler. *Thorax* 1995; 51: 985–988.

19. Pierart F, Wildhaber JH, Vrancken I, *et al*. Washing plastic spacers in household detergent reduces electrostatic charge and greatly improves delivery. *Eur Respir J* 1999; 13: 673–678.

20. British Thoracic Society/Scottish Intercollegiate Guidelines Network. British Guideline on the Management of Asthma. *Thorax* 2003; 58 (Suppl I): S1–S94.

21. Cochrane GM. Compliance and outcomes in patients with asthma. *Drugs* 1996; 52 (Suppl 6): 12–19.

22. Mann M, Eliasson O, Patel K, *et al*. A comparison of the effects of bid and qid dosing on compliance with inhaled flunisolide. *Chest* 1992; 101: 496–499.

23. Blake KV, Harman E, Hendeles L. Evaluation of a generic albuterol metered dose inhaler: importance of priming the MDI. *Ann Allergy* 1992; 62: 169–174.

24. British Thoracic Society Nebuliser Project Group. Current best practice for nebuliser treatment. *Thorax* 1997; 52 (Suppl 2).

25. Kassner F, Hodder R, Bateman ED. A review of ipratropium bromide/fenoterol hydrobromide (Berodual) delivered via Respimat Soft Mist Inhaler in patients with asthma and chronic obstructive pulmonary disease. *Drugs* 2004; 64: 1671–1682.

26. Chan H-K, Chew NYK. Novel alternative methods for the delivery of drugs for the treatment of asthma. *Adv Drug Deliv Rev* 2003; 55: 793–805.
27. Gonda I, Schuster JA, Rubsamen RM. Inhalation delivery systems with compliance and disease management capabilities. *J Controlled Release* 1998; 53: 269–274.
28. Farr SJ, Rowe AM, Rubsamen R, *et al.* Aerosol deposition in the human lung following administration from a microprocessor controlled pressurised metered dose inhaler. *Thorax* 1995; 50: 639–644.

8

Patient education and self-management

Patient education

Patient education is an essential component of the management of asthma, the goal being to improve asthma control by improving knowledge and changing behaviour. Providing patients with information should empower them to take part in decision making and to undertake self-management of their disease appropriately and effectively. Studies have shown that well-informed patients with asthma are more able to manage their condition and have better health-related outcomes.[1] Indeed, concordance with medications and adherence to advice offered by the health professional depend on the patient's understanding of the nature of the disease as well as the benefits of self-management and satisfaction with the information provided.[1,2]

Information provided should be tailored to the individual patient's needs. Different approaches are needed depending on social, emotional and disease status, as well according to the patient's age and level of education.[3]

The need for health professionals to offer patients high-quality and accessible information is increasingly being recognised within the NHS. It is important that health professionals who have contact with patients are well trained and offer uniform, evidence-based advice to the patient. Nothing unsettles a patient more than receiving apparently conflicting messages from various health professionals. The British Thoracic Society /Scottish Intercollegiate Guidelines Network (BTS/SIGN) asthma guideline is an excellent tool for good management and is available to all health professionals.[3] However, guidelines alone are not sufficient to deliver uniform patient education; there needs to be adequate dissemination and implementation of their content.

It is important to remember that even if the health professional does an excellent job in educating the patient, a knowledgeable patient does not automatically use that knowledge to alter their behaviour or their attitude towards an illness.[4] Patients are subject to numerous outside influences, such as the media, family and peers, which may provide the patient with conflicting information, leading to confusion. Furthermore, there are a number of barriers to providing good patient education, related to the patient, disease and medication (see Management Focus, below).

It is estimated that 40–80% of medical information provided by health professionals is forgotten immediately. The greater the amount of information presented, the lower the proportion correctly recalled.[5] Furthermore, almost half of the information that is remembered is incorrect.[6] Reinforcement of the message on subsequent occasions is therefore essential. By the time the patient has heard the same information three times, retention rate approaches 100%.

Written information

The verbal message can be reinforced by providing supplementary written information. Many leaflets for patients with asthma are available. These should be used as part of the consultation between patient and health professional; simply giving written information alone is unlikely to alter a patient's behaviour. Written information should be used as an adjunct to, not a substitute for, verbal communication.

MANAGEMENT FOCUS

Potential barriers to patient education	
Disease barriers	Misconceptions about the nature of the condition
Psychological barriers	Denial and disbelief of diagnosis
	Uncertainty and feelings of 'not being in control'
	Conflicting messages from outside influences, such as the media and family
	Apparently conflicting messages from health professionals
	Feelings of stigmatisation
	Depression
	'It won't happen to me'
Medication-related barriers	Drugs cause side-effects
	Distrust of all medications
	Dislike of dependency
	Belief that bronchodilators are best
	'Steroid phobia'

It is important to consider the quality of the written information, as this varies considerably. A review of UK-based asthma leaflets used in general practice found that many had an inappropriately high readability score and many contained inaccurate information.[7] It is worth bearing in mind that much of the reading matter encountered in adult life is roughly equivalent to GCSE pass level, and yet almost half of the adult population in the UK do not have reading skills at this level. Poor health and poor basic skills (i.e. numeracy and literacy skills) often go hand in hand. Patients can go to great lengths to disguise problems (e.g. by 'forgetting' their reading glasses or bringing a family member to a consultation) and health professionals are largely unaware of the extent of the problem in the general population.

Much of the information obtained from the Internet is pitched at a high readability level. The quality and accuracy of information is highly variable[8] and much is promotional or from overseas, providing potentially conflicting advice. It is always advisable to use and refer patients to credible websites (see Management Focus, page 136). Asthma UK (formerly the National Asthma Campaign) provides high-quality non-promotional information. The Global Initiative for Asthma (GINA) provides educational materials for patients whose first language is not English. Remember, however, that not all individuals who speak another language can read it (including native English speakers). Family members are often used as translators but this can present problems with confidentiality and accuracy. Bilingual link workers should be used where possible.

Timing

The timing of when information is given is important. Often it is given at or near the time of diagnosis. For some people this can be a distressing and confusing time and they may not be ready to receive information about their illness.[9] Some patients may feel overwhelmed by the volume of information provided in one consultation. There are many opportunities to provide information: at review clinics, in the community pharmacy and at emergency attendances and hospital admissions.[3] Unfortunately, these tend not be exploited because of time constraints. The recommendation in the BTS/SIGN guideline on asthma management is to provide "brief, simple education, linked to patient goals". The communication of information to patients need not be prolonged to be effective.

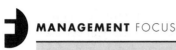

MANAGEMENT FOCUS

Sources of information for patients and health professionals

For patients and health professionals

Asthma UK (formerly National Asthma Campaign)
www.asthma.org.uk

Asthma UK England
Summit House, 70 Wilson Street, London EC2A 2DB
Tel: 020 7786 4900   Queries about asthma: 08457 010203
Email: info@asthma.org.uk

Asthma UK Scotland
4 Queen Street, Edinburgh EH2 1JE.
Tel: 0131 226 2544
Email: scotland@asthma.org.uk

Asthma UK Cymru
3rd floor, Eastgate House, 34–43 Newport Road, Cardiff CF24 0AB
Tel: 02920 435 400
Email: wales@asthma.org.uk

Asthma UK Northern Ireland
Peace House, 224 Lisburn Road, Belfast BT9 6GE
Tel: 02890 669736
Email: ni@asthma.org.uk

Mainly for patients

British Lung Foundation
73–75 Goswell Road, London EC1V 7ER
www.lunguk.org
Tel: 08458 50 50 20

NHS Direct
Tel: 0845 4647

Allergy UK (formerly British Allergy Foundation)
3 White Oak Square, London Road, Swanley, Kent BR8 7AG
www.allergyuk.org
Allergy Helpline: 01322 619898
E-mail: info@allergyuk.org

Mainly for health professionals

Education for Health (formerly National Respiratory Training Centre)
The Athenaeum, 10 Church Street, Warwick CV34 4AB
www.educationforhealth.org.uk
Tel: 01926 493313
Email: enquiries@educationforhealth.org.uk

General Practice Airways Group (GPIAG)
Smithy House, Waterbeck, Lockerbie DG11 3EY
www.gpiag.org.uk
Tel: 01461 600639
Email: info@gpiag.org

British Thoracic Society (BTS)
17 Doughty Street, London WC1N 2PL
www.brit-thoracic.org.uk
Tel: 020 7831 8778
Email: bts@brit-thoracic.org.uk

How much information?

Interestingly, it has been reported that asthma patients want more information than they currently receive.[10,11] One study showed that only 45% of patients were satisfied with the amount of information they had.[12] The BTS/SIGN guideline provides a list of the minimum information that should be provided to patients with asthma (see Management Focus, page 138).[3] The list is intended to be used as a framework that health professionals can adapt to meet the needs of individual patients or carers. It is important to identify the patient's own education needs and it is worthwhile to encourage patients to think in advance about questions they might have. Individualised approaches to information giving are more efficacious than generalised ones.[13]

Education is a process

The best result from patient education is thus achieved from the development of a partnership between patient (or parent/carer) and health professional, in which communication is of the highest standard and where treatment advice is individualised for that patient and backed up with written information. The patient will need to be reviewed regularly and messages reinforced. It is important to recognise that education is a process, not a single event.

Self-management

Many deaths from asthma in the UK occur before admission to hospital and thus before administration of appropriate drugs is possible. The key to managing an acute asthma attack and reducing asthma mortality is

MANAGEMENT FOCUS

Topics to be addressed with patients or parents/carers: the minimum information that should be provided to patients with asthma according to the asthma management guideline published by the British Thoracic Society/Scottish Intercollegiate Guidelines Network[3]

Nature of the disease

- Chronic but treatable disease
- Appropriate allergen or trigger avoidance

Nature of the treatment

- Rationale for the use of bronchodilators and anti-inflammatory drugs
- Reasons for regular medication and follow-up

How to use treatments

- Instruction on the use of an inhaler
- Instruction on use of a peak flow meter for monitoring

Development of self-monitoring/self-assessment skills

- Negotiation of the asthma action plan in light of identified patient goals
- Recognition and management of acute exacerbations
- Steps to take when deterioration occurs

for the patient to recognise deteriorating symptoms and to initiate treatment promptly. This self-management approach therefore involves the patient managing their own treatment rather than consulting a doctor or nurse before making changes. The BTS/SIGN guideline recommends that the majority of patients with asthma should have an agreed written action plan (self-management plan) that instructs them on how to recognise and react to acute attacks and when to summon help.[3] Patient education and simple action plans can reduce hospital admissions, visits to general practitioners and mortality in both adults and children.

Self-management education has been compared with routine care in over 36 randomised controlled trials. Systematic review of these studies shows that self-medication leads to a 40% reduction in hospitalisations, 20% reduction in visits to emergency departments and improvements in night-time symptoms and time off work and school. In other words, self-management impacts positively on all aspects of disease burden. The evidence is particularly good for patients in secondary care with moderate-to-severe asthma, and those who have had recent exacerbations.

The limited number of primary care studies show less consistent results, perhaps because clinical benefit is harder to demonstrate in patients with mild asthma. A consistent finding in many studies has been improvement in patient outcomes, such as self-efficacy (the belief in one's abilities to produce a certain outcome or goal), knowledge and confidence.[1,2,14,15] Considering the overwhelming evidence for the effectiveness of self-management plans, it is astonishing that few patients have a written plan in place. Although most action plans are set up and delivered by trained asthma health professionals, usually doctors and nurses, they often resist implementing the plans, being unconvinced of the benefits and unwilling to devote extra time on the consultation. It is true that extra time is required to write and develop the plan and to provide supporting education. However, investment of time early on is likely to be paid back in the long term, as self-management education has been shown to reduce unscheduled consultations with general practitioners.[1] Trying to reduce the workload by removing the education component of the plan is not recommended, as previous work shows that plans which do not provide education are unlikely to be successful.

Individualising the plan according to the patient's asthma severity, needs and personal objectives (e.g. wanting to be able to sleep better at night) is more effective than using generalised plans. Different approaches to self-management may be required to suit different patients. Innovative approaches to self-management education in teenagers (web-based, peer-delivered within schools) appear to have been more success than traditional programmes. A different approach may be needed for children under 5 years of age, many of whom have viral-induced wheeze. There are no studies that specifically address the provision of self-management education for the elderly.

Every consultation with a patient with asthma is an opportunity to review the patient's self-management skills. Certainly no patient should leave hospital after an acute exacerbation without a written action plan or without having had their action plan reviewed and updated. An acute exacerbation offers an opportunity to investigate how the patient dealt with their deteriorating symptoms and to offer further advice.

Self-management programmes will only achieve better health outcomes if the asthma treatment prescribed is appropriate and within guideline recommendations. There is some evidence that patients who are provided with an asthma action plan receive more effective treatment.

The action plan

Patients prefer the term 'action plan' rather than 'self-management plan' as it appears less daunting. It can also be used when working with parents and carers as well as with adult patients.

The recognition of deteriorating asthma requires interpretation of both subjective and objective measures of asthma severity. In practice, self-monitoring is based on symptoms, peak flow measurements or both depending on the patient's preference or ability (see Chapter 6). The inability of a patient to appreciate the severity of an attack may lead to a delay in seeking appropriate medical attention. Studies have identified key observations that indicate significant worsening of asthma to the patient. In particular, the development of nocturnal asthma is recognised as a good marker of unstable asthma, as is a poor response to the increased use of short-acting beta-2 agonists. Peak flow meters measure the degree of airflow obstruction. The patient records their personal-best peak flow measurement, providing an objective baseline against which to gauge any subsequent deterioration in asthma control. Subsequent asthma exacerbations are then most easily interpreted by patients when expressed as a percentage of this personal-best value. The written action plan should inform patients about when and how to modify medications in response to worsening asthma and how and when to access the medical system in response to worsening asthma.

Home action plans should include the following:

- instructions on how to recognise signs of worsening asthma
- advice on the prompt use of short-acting beta-2 agonists and oral corticosteroids
- monitoring of response to medications
- contact information/telephone numbers
- follow-up to assess asthma control.

A number of educational tools are available to support health professionals, many of which are free, well researched and non-promotional. Amongst these are the *Be in Control* materials produced by Asthma UK (formerly the National Asthma Campaign), accessible from the website (www.asthma.org.uk) or by contacting the organisation (see Management Focuses on pages 136, 141 and 142).

An example of an action plan based on a patient with a personal-best peak expiratory flow (PEF) of 500 litres/minute

Symptoms are:	PEF is:	Action is:
• No asthma symptoms during the day or night • No asthma symptoms whilst undertaking normal activities	500 litres/minute >85% of best (i.e. >425 litres/minute)	• Normal – asthma under control • Continue to take your usual asthma medications • Talk to your nurse/doctor/pharmacist about taking less treatment if your asthma is always under control
• Symptoms during day and/or night • Difficulty sleeping because of your asthma • Needing to use reliever inhaler more than once a day	<425 litre/minute 70–85% of best	• Take two puffs twice a day of steroid inhaler • Use blue inhaler for relief of symptoms • It is important to take your steroid inhaler regularly as directed
• Out of breath • Symptoms all the time • Blue inhaler does not work	<350 litres/minute 50–75% of best	• Continue on above medications • Start steroid tablets: prednisolone tablets 40–50 mg every morning • Contact general practitioner
• Too breathless to speak	<250 litres/minute <50% of best	• Go to hospital emergency department or call for ambulance immediately

Example of a personal asthma action plan (Asthma UK)

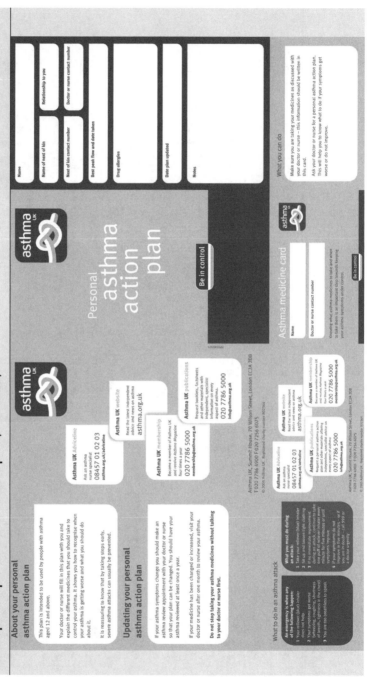

Zone 1

Your asthma is under control if:

- You have no or minimal symptoms during the day or night (wheezing, coughing, shortness of breath, tightness in the chest)
- You can do all of your normal activities without asthma symptoms
- Your peak flow reading is above [ ] (85% of your best)

Action

Continue to take your usual asthma medicines.

Preventer medicine should be used every day, even when you are feeling well. Your preventer medicine is

name [ ]

colour [ ] Take [ ] number of puffs/doses

dosage [ ]

when [ ]

Reliever medicine should be used if you have symptoms. Your reliever medicine is

name [ ]

colour [ ] Take [ ] number of puffs/doses

when [ ]

Other medicines taken regularly may be added to your treatment if your preventer is not stopping all of your symptoms. Your add-on medicine is name [ ]

colour [ ] Take [ ] number of puffs/doses

when [ ]

If you are always in zone 1, your doctor or nurse may want to reduce (step down) your regular medicines.

Zone 2

Your asthma gets worse if:

- You need to use your reliever inhaler more than once a day
- You have had difficulty sleeping because of your asthma
- Your peak flow reading is between [ ] and [ ] (between 70% and 85% of your best)

Action

Increase your preventer inhaler

name [ ]

colour [ ] Take [ ] number of puffs/doses

dosage [ ] when [ ]

Stay on this dose until you have had no symptoms for [ ] days then return to your usual dose in zone 1.

Continue to take your reliever medicine

name [ ]

colour [ ] when [ ] when needed.

If your symptoms do not improve in [ ] days contact your doctor or nurse for advice.

Your doctor or nurse will discuss your inhaler with you and check your inhaler technique. You may be started on a different medicine to help you get your symptoms back under control.

If you are often in zone 2, let your doctor or nurse know at your next review. Your usual medicines may need to be increased or changed.

Zone 3

Your asthma is much more severe if:

- You need to take your reliever inhaler every four hours or more often
- You have symptoms all the time
- Your peak flow reading is between [ ] and [ ] (between 50% and 70% of your best)

Action

Continue taking your preventer medicine as prescribed at the higher dose in zone 2.

Continue to take your reliever medicine when needed.

If you have been prescribed steroid tablets, take

number [ ] 5mg prednisolone

tablets immediately and again every morning for [ ] days or until your symptoms have improved or your peak flow has been at [ ] for two days.

Your doctor or nurse may want you tu let them know within 24–36 hours that you have started a course of steroid tablets. If you regularly take steroid tablets, your doctor or nurse will advise you on how to reduce the number you are taking.

If you are often in zone 3, let your doctor or nurse know. Your usual medicines may need to be increased or changed.

Zone 4

It is an asthma emergency if any of the following happen:

1 Your reliever (blue) inhaler does not help
2 Your symptoms get worse (cough, breathless, wheeze, tight chest)
3 You are too breathless to speak
4 Your peak flow reading is below [ ]

Action

1 Take your reliever (blue) inhaler

2 Sit up and loosen tight clothing

3 If no immediate improvement during an attack, continue to take one puff/dose of reliever inhaler every minute for five minutes or until symptoms improve

4 If your symptoms do not improve in five minutes – or if you are in doubt – call 999 or a doctor urgently

How to recognise if your asthma is getting worse

Have you had difficulty sleeping because of your asthma symptoms (including coughing)?

Have you had your usual asthma symptoms during the day (wheezing, coughing, shortness of breath, tightness in the chest)?

Has your asthma interfered with your usual activities (eg housework, work or school)?

If **'yes'** to one or more of the above, or if you have not seen your doctor or nurse about your asthma for 12 months or more, arrange to have a review. If **'yes'** to all of the above – is this an emergency? (see overleaf)

Your asthma medicines – what to use on an everyday basis

	Your medicine is:	How much to use:	When to use:	Comments/symptoms:
Preventer				
Reliever				
Other				

References

1. Gibson PG, Coughlan J, Wilson AJ, *et al*. Self-management education and regular practitioner review for adults with asthma (Cochrane Review). *The Cochrane Library*, issue 3. Chichester: John Wiley & Sons, 2001 (*www.the cochranelibrary.com*).
2. Gibson PG, Coughlan J, Wilson AJ, *et al*. The effects of self-management education and regular practitioner review in adults with asthma. (Cochrane Review). *The Cochrane Library*, issue 4. Chichester: John Wiley & Sons, 1998 (*www.thecochranelibrary.com*).
3. British Thoracic Society/Scottish Intercollegiate Guidelines Network. British Guideline on the Management of Asthma. *Thorax* 2003; 58 (Suppl I): S1–S94.
4. Horne R, Weinman J. Self-regulation and self-management in asthma: exploring the role of illness perceptions and treatment beliefs in explaining non-adherence to preventer medication. *Psychol Health* 2002; 17: 17–32.
5. McGuire LC. Remembering what the doctor said: organisation and older adults' memory for medical information. *Exp Aging Res* 1996; 22: 403–428.
6. Kessels RPC. Patients' memory for medical intervention. *J R Soc Med* 2003; 96: 219–222.
7. Smith H, Gooding S, Brown R, *et al*. Evaluation of readability and accuracy of information leaflets in general practice for patients with asthma. *BMJ* 1998; 317: 264–265.
8. Croft DR, Peterson MW. An evaluation of the quality and contents of asthma education on the World Wide Web. *Chest* 2002; 121: 1301–1308.
9. Caress A, Luker KA, Woodcock A, *et al*. An exploratory study of priority information needs in adult asthma patients. *Patient Ed Counsel* 2002; 47: 319–327.
10. Koning CJM, Maille AR, Stevens I, *et al*. Patients' opinions on respiratory care: do doctors fulfill their needs? *J Asthma* 1995; 32: 355–363.
11. Partridge MR. Asthma: lessons from patient education. *Patient Educ Counsel* 1995; 26: 81–86.
12. Caress A, Beaver K, Luker K, *et al*. A cross sectional survey of priority information needs in adult asthma patients. *Am J Respir Crit Care Med* 2002; 165: A43.
13. Thoonen BPA, Schermer TRJ, Jansen M, *et al*. Asthma education tailored to individual patient needs can optimise partnerships in asthma self management. *Patient Educ Counsel* 2002; 47: 355–360.
14. Partridge MR. Self-management in adults with asthma. *Patient Educ Counsel* 1997; 32: 1–4.
15. Lahdensuo A, Haahtela T, Herrala J, *et al*. Randomised comparison of guided self-management and traditional treatment of asthma over one year. *BMJ* 1996; 312: 748–752.

9

Asthma in pregnancy

Several physiological changes occur during pregnancy that could worsen or improve asthma[1] (see Monitoring Focus, below). For example, hormonal changes in pregnancy affect the upper respiratory tract and the airway mucosa, leading to mucosal oedema and hypersecretion. Also, as the uterus enlarges during pregnancy, there is an elevation of the diaphragm. Diaphragm function is not impaired but there is an associated change in pulmonary function. Pregnancy can affect the course of asthma and asthma can affect pregnancy outcomes.

Effects of pregnancy on asthma

In a prospective cohort study of 366 pregnancies in 330 asthmatic women, asthma worsened in 35% of cases.[2] Studies from the United

 MONITORING FOCUS

Physiological changes in pregnancy[1]	
Measure	**Change**
Pulmonary function tests	
Forced expiratory volume	No change
Peak expiratory flow	No change or decreased
Respiration rate	No change or slightly increased
Tidal volume	Increased by 30–35%
Arterial blood gases	
pH	No change
$PaCO_2$	Decreased
PaO_2	Increased
Serum bicarbonate concentration	Decreased

PaO_2, arterial oxygen tension; $PaCO_2$, arterial carbon dioxide tension.

States suggest that 11–18% of pregnant women with asthma will have at least one visit to the emergency department for acute asthma; of these, 62% will require hospitalisation.[3] Generally, about one-third of women with asthma experience an improvement in their asthma during pregnancy, one-third experience a worsening of symptoms and in one-third symptoms remain the same.[3] The course of asthma during pregnancy is generally unpredictable but there is some evidence that it is similar in successive pregnancies.[2]

There have been some general observations on the effects of pregnancy on asthma. The peak increase in asthma symptoms during pregnancy occurs between 24 and 36 weeks' gestation. In the last 4 weeks of pregnancy, asthma symptoms lessen in comparison with any other gestational period.[2] Moreover, increased severity of asthma during labour is rare if asthma control is maintained during pregnancy. In a large cohort study, 90% of women had no asthma symptoms during labour or delivery. Of those who did, only two required more treatment than standard inhaled bronchodilators.[2]

Effects of asthma on pregnancy

Uncontrolled asthma is associated with many maternal and fetal complications, including preterm birth, low-birth-weight infants, increased perinatal mortality, pre-eclampsia, hyperemesis, vaginal haemorrhage, intrauterine growth restriction, neonatal hypoxia and a higher rate of emergency caesarean section.[3] In contrast, if asthma is well controlled throughout pregnancy, there is little or no increased risk of maternal or fetal complications. Pregnant women should therefore have their treatments optimised and their lung function maximised to reduce the risk of exacerbations. The risks to the mother and fetus of uncontrolled acute or under-treated asthma far outweigh any risks from using asthma medications.

Asthma management during pregnancy

Asthma management during pregnancy is similar to that in non-pregnant adults (see Chapter 3).[3] The goals of asthma therapy during pregnancy are to deliver a healthy infant, optimise airway function and maintain normal activity levels, control symptoms, avoid adverse effects of medication and to prevent an acute asthma exacerbation. If an asthma exacerbation occurs during pregnancy, the patient should receive drug therapy as for a non-pregnant patient with acute asthma (see Chapter 4). The principal goal of treating an exacerbation should be the control of hypoxia. Oxygen should be delivered to maintain oxygen saturation above 95% in order to prevent maternal and fetal hypoxia. Early intervention during acute exacerbations is a key factor to the prevention of impaired maternal–fetal oxygenation.

Patient education is critical to successful asthma management and should be initiated before pregnancy. Education should include continued concordance with medication regimens, reassurance regarding the safety of medicines in pregnancy, and methods to monitor pulmonary function at home using peak expiratory flow rate. Factors that trigger the woman's asthma should be identified and avoided to help asthma control. However, routine skin-prick testing for allergens during pregnancy is not recommended because there is a slight risk of anaphylaxis in some patients. Special attention needs to be made to smoking cessation and to controlling gastro-oesophageal reflux, as both can improve the control of asthma during pregnancy.

Pharmacological therapy in pregnancy

In general, the medicines used to treat asthma are safe in pregnancy.[3,4] However, it is good practice to consider a number of points before prescribing for pregnant women with asthma (see Management Focus, page 148).

No significant association has been demonstrated between major congenital malformations or adverse perinatal outcome and exposure to beta-2 agonists (e.g. salbutamol),[5] inhaled steroids[4] or methylxanthines.[4,6] Evidence from prescription event monitoring suggests that salmeterol is also safe in pregnancy.[7] Ipratropium bromide appears to be safe in pregnancy and is helpful in acute asthma exacerbations when given in conjunction with beta-2 agonists. Congenital abnormalities, such as cleft palate, have been reported in animals given high doses of systemic corticosteroids in the first trimester[8] but data from many studies in humans have failed to demonstrate this association and the balance of evidence suggests that steroid tablets are not teratogenic.[4,9,10] Even if the association is real, the benefit of steroids to the mother and the fetus for a life-threatening disease justifies their use in pregnancy. If an exacerbation is left untreated, the risks to both the mother and fetus are far greater. In practice, oral corticosteroids are not given as freely to pregnant women with asthma as to non-pregnant women but steroid tablets should never be withheld because of pregnancy.

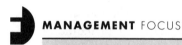

Recommendations for prescribing during pregnancy

- Offer pre-pregnancy counselling to women with asthma regarding the importance and safety of continuing their asthma medications during pregnancy to ensure good asthma control.
- Monitor pregnant women with asthma closely so that any change in course can be matched with an appropriate change in treatment.
- Give drug therapy for acute asthma as for the non-pregnant patient.
- Use beta-2 agonists, inhaled steroids and oral and intravenous theophylline as normal during pregnancy.
- Check blood levels of theophylline in patients with acute severe asthma and in those critically dependent on therapeutic theophylline levels. Protein binding decreases in pregnancy, resulting in increased free drug and higher blood levels.
- Use steroid tablets as normal when indicated during pregnancy for severe asthma. Steroid tablets should never be withheld because of pregnancy.
- Do not start leukotriene antagonists during pregnancy. They may be continued in women who, before pregnancy, have demonstrated significant improvement in asthma control with these agents that was not achievable with other medications.

Safety data relating to the two leukotriene receptor antagonists currently available in the UK for the treatment of asthma (montelukast and zafirlukast) is limited but animal studies and post-marketing surveillance data are reassuring. The current recommendation is to not commence leukotriene receptor antagonists during pregnancy but they may be continued in women who have demonstrated significant improvements in asthma control with these agents before pregnancy which was not achievable with other medications.[3]

Labour and delivery

As mentioned above, acute asthma attacks during labour and delivery are rare. During labour, endogenous steroids are produced which are thought to help control the disease. If the patient has received steroid tablets at a dose exceeding prednisolone 7.5 mg daily for more than 2 weeks before delivery, intravenous hydrocortisone 100 mg 6–8 hourly should be administered during labour. Prostaglandin E2 can be used safely to induce labour, whereas prostaglandin F2α should be avoided as it can induce bronchospasm, particularly in association with general anaesthesia. Although ergometrine has been reported to cause bronchospasm, this has not been associated with administration of Syntometrine and thus this is the treatment choice for prophylaxis against postpartum haemorrhage.

Women with asthma may safely use all forms of pain relief in labour. However, epidural anaesthesia is preferred to general anaesthesia in women with asthma because it reduces oxygen consumption during labour. Women should be advised to continue to use their usual asthma medications during labour.

The post-partum period

Altered control of asthma during pregnancy usually reverts back to a pre-pregnancy state within 3 months of delivery.

Breastfeeding

The Department of Health supports advice from the World Health Organization for mothers to breastfeed exclusively until the child is 6 months old. Breastfeeding should be encouraged, and medications that are considered safe during pregnancy can be administered during breastfeeding. Theophylline is generally well-tolerated, although there have been reports of it causing irritability and jitteriness. Prednisolone is secreted into breast milk, but concentrations are only 5–25% of those in the mother's serum;[11] consequently, low-to-moderate doses of prednisolone (<40 mg daily) are unlikely to cause effects on the infant. If the mother is taking a higher dose, the recommendation is that she should allow 4 hours before breastfeeding, and the infant should be monitored for adrenal suppression. In practice, however, it may be difficult to allow 4 hours between a dose of corticosteroid and breastfeeding, as newborns in particular usually require more frequent feeds. A good option is to express breastmilk for this one feed. The inhaled route of administration should be recommended where possible because, as a general rule, inhaled medications have a low systemic absorption and are well-tolerated.

Asthma is an atopic condition and it has been suggested that breastfeeding can protect an infant from developing atopy, although there is no evidence that clearly supports or refutes this. The evidence suggests that if there is a strong family history of atopy, breastfeeding will be beneficial; where there is no atopy in the family, however, it might delay the onset of atopy but does not reduce the prevalence.[12]

References

1. Elkus R, Popovich J. Respiratory physiology in pregnancy. *Clin Chest Med* 1992; 13: 555–565.
2. Schatz M, Harden K, Forsythe A, *et al.* The course of asthma during pregnancy, post partum and with successive pregnancies: a prospective analysis. *J Allergy Clin Immunol* 1998; 81: 509–517.
3. British Thoracic Society/Scottish Intercollegiate Guidelines Network. British Guideline on the Management of Asthma. *Thorax* 2003; 58 (Suppl I): S1–S94.
4. Schatz M, Zeiger RS, Harden K, *et al.* The safety of asthma and allergy medications during pregnancy. *J Allergy Clin Immunol* 1997; 100: 301–306.
5. Schatz M, Zeiger RS, Harden K, *et al.* The safety of inhaled beta-agonist bronchodilators during pregnancy. *J Allergy Clin Immunol* 1988; 82: 686–695.
6. Stenius-Aarniala B, Riikonrn S, Teramo K. Slow-release theophylline in pregnant asthmatics. *Chest* 1995; 107: 642–647.
7. Mann RD, Kubota K, Pearce G, *et al.* Salmeterol: a study by prescription event monitoring in a UK cohort of 15,407 patients. *J Clin Epidemiol* 1996; 49: 247–250.
8. Fainstat T. Cortisol induced congenital cleft palate in rabbits. *Endocrinology* 1964; 55: 502–511.
9. Fitzimmons R, Greenberger PA, Patterson R. Outcomes of pregnancy in women requiring corticosteroids for severe asthma. *J Allergy Clin Immunol* 1986; 78: 349–353.
10. Czeizel AE, Rockenbauer M. Population-based case-control study of teratogenic potential of corticosteroids. *Teratology* 1997; 56: 335–340.
11. Ost L, Wettrell G, Bjorkhem I, *et al.* Prednisolone excretion in human milk. *Arch Dis Child* 1975; 50: 894–896.
12. Luyt D. Breastfeeding: Is it protective against atopy? *Airways J* 2004; 2: 149–151.

10

Beta-2 agonists

Indications

Beta-2 agonists are widely used to relieve bronchoconstriction. In addition to an acute bronchodilator effect, they protect against various challenges, such as exercise, cold air and allergen. They are the bronchodilators of choice in treating acute severe asthma.

- Salbutamol and terbutaline are indicated to relieve symptoms on an as-required basis for all patients with asthma.
- Salmeterol and formoterol are selective long-acting inhaled beta-2 agonists indicated for regular treatment at step 3 and above of the British Thoracic Society/Scottish Intercollegiate Guidelines Network (BTS/SIGN) asthma management guideline.[1] Salmeterol and formoterol should be added to existing corticosteroid therapy, not replace it. They should not be used for the relief of an acute asthma attack.

Mechanism of action

The majority of the beta-2 agonists currently used in asthma are structurally related to adrenaline. The chemical structures of some of these agents are illustrated in Figure 10.1.

Beta-2 agonists are sympathomimetic bronchodilators. They produce bronchodilation by directly stimulating beta-2 adrenoceptors in airway smooth muscle, mimicking the effects of the sympathetic nervous system. Salbutamol is hydrophilic and interacts directly with the beta-2-adrenoceptors from the aqueous phase.[2] In contrast, salmeterol is lipophilic and initially associates predominately with the lipid bilayer of the cell membrane, followed by membrane translocation. This indirect binding delays the onset of action of salmeterol.[3] Formoterol is partially lipophilic; its action is more rapid in onset than that of salmeterol.

Activation of beta-2 adrenoceptors results in activation of adenyl cyclase, leading to an increase in intracellular cyclic 3,5-adenosine monophosphate (cAMP). This results in activation of a specific kinase

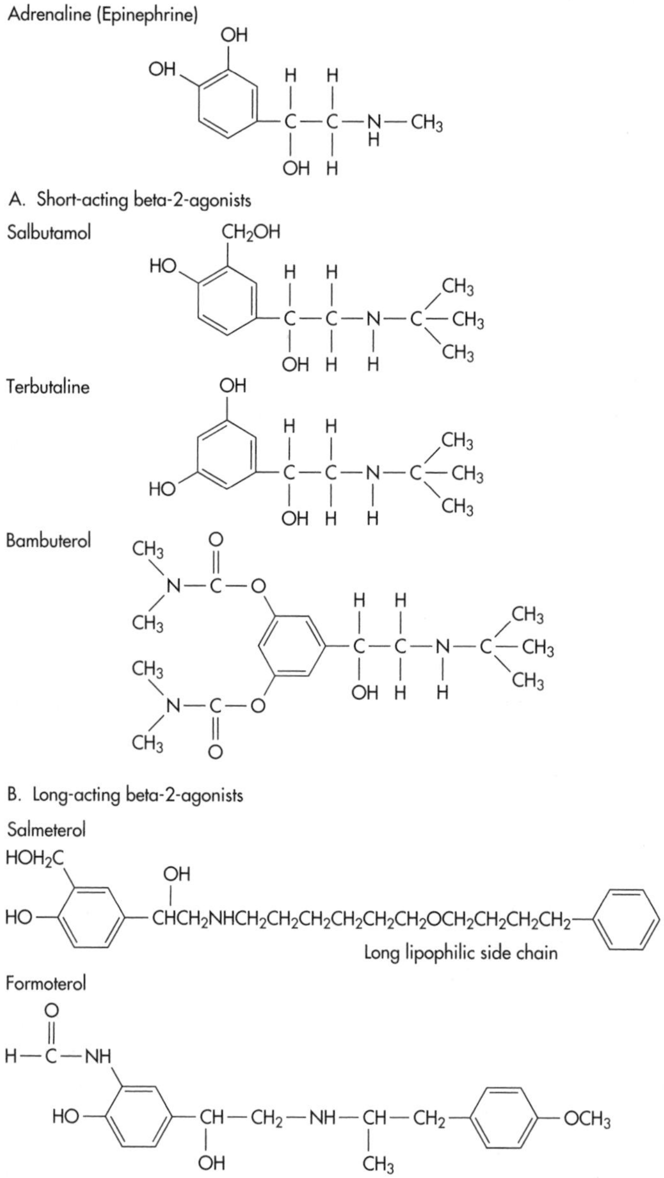

Figure 10.1 Chemical structures of adrenaline (epinephrine) and currently used short- and long-acting beta-2 agonists.

(protein kinase A) that phosphorylates several target proteins within the cell. The phosphorylation process leads to muscle relaxation by several processes:

- lowering of the raised intracellular calcium ion concentration associated with muscle contraction by active uptake of calcium ions from the cell into intracellular stores
- inhibition of phosphoinositide hydrolysis, reducing the cystolic free calcium concentration
- direct inhibition of myosin light chain kinase, preventing the molecular interaction of myosin with actin and contraction of the smooth muscle
- opening of large-conductance calcium-activated potassium channels that repolarise the smooth muscle cell.

The overall effect is relaxation of the smooth muscle tone and a reduction in the dynamic hyperinflation, which together provide rapid relief of symptoms and an improved exercise tolerance.

Beta-2 agonists may have many additional effects on airways:

- reduced plasma exudation
- there is some evidence that beta-2 agonists increase mucociliary clearance in patients with asthma[4]
- beta-2 agonists are potent mast-cell stabilisers, suggesting that they may modify inflammation, although this effect is probably of minimal clinical significance; interestingly, this effect appears to relate only to acute inflammation – beta-2 agonists do not have any significant inhibitory effect on chronic inflammation
- beta-2 agonists may reduce adherence of bacteria to airway epithelial cells, which may reduce the severity of infectious exacerbations.[5]

Pharmacological properties

Short-acting beta-2 agonists (salbutamol, terbutaline) relax bronchial smooth muscle and cause a rapid increase in airflow. They are the most potent and rapidly acting (within 3–5 minutes) bronchodilators available. The bronchodilator effects usually wear off within 4–6 hours.

The long-acting beta-2 agonists, salmeterol and formoterol, have different pharmacology. They both cause bronchodilation for at least 12 hours after a single administration, but formoterol has an almost immediate onset of action (3–5 minutes) while that of salmeterol is delayed by 15–30 minutes. Only formoterol is licensed for administration on an as-needed basis.[6] The dose of formoterol is more flexible than that of salmeterol, which cannot be increased because of adverse effects. Lower doses of long-acting beta-2 agonists are equally effective in most patients and should be tried first. The optimal dose of salmeterol for patients with mild or moderate asthma is 50 micrograms twice daily (this dose provides similar efficacy but fewer side-effects than 100 micrograms twice daily). The higher dose has been shown to be more effective in controlling PEF and asthma symptoms in patients with severe asthma who are taking oral corticosteroids who do not respond adequately to the 50 microgram dose. Formoterol shows a linear dose–response relationship up to 54 micrograms daily.

The pharmacological properties of the beta-2 agonists are summarised in Table 10.1.

Route of administration

Beta-2 agonists can be administered by inhalation, orally or parenterally. The inhaled route is preferred, as the drug reaches the lungs directly, producing a faster onset of action and fewer systemic side-effects. The oral route can be used for patients who cannot manage the inhaled route, although this is a rare occurrence. Slow-release oral beta-2 agonist preparations (e.g. bambuterol and slow-release salbutamol) are not routinely advocated to treat asthma: although these preparations may treat peripheral airways more effectively, the onset of action is slower and there are more side-effects than with inhaled preparations. Bambuterol (see Figure 10.1) is a prodrug that is slowly hydrolysed to terbutaline in the plasma by cholinesterases; metabolism occurs in the liver and possibly in lung tissue. Stable terbutaline plasma levels and adequate bronchodilation for 24 hours have been reported with once-daily doses of bambuterol. The elimination half-life of terbutaline after bambuterol administration is extended to approximately 20 hours. Bambuterol appears to be as effective as twice-daily inhaled salmeterol.[7,8]

Salbutamol and terbutaline can be given by intravenous infusion for severe asthma (see Chapter 4). These drugs can also be administered via the subcutaneous route on a regular basis but this is not recommended. The evidence of benefit is uncertain and adverse effects limit the dose that can be given.

Tables 10.2 and 10.3 summarise the dosages and indications of the short- and long-acting beta-2-agonists.

Combination products

Over the last 5 years prescribing of corticosteroids as single preparations has decreased in favour of prescribing combination preparations. Combination inhalers contain fixed doses of a long-acting beta-2 agonist and an inhaled corticosteroid. The rationale for giving a long-acting beta-2 agonist and corticosteroid together is based on a beneficial interaction

Table 10.1 Properties of beta-2 agonists

	Salbutamol	Terbutaline	Formoterol	Salmeterol
Potency	Moderately potent	Moderately potent	Very potent	Potent
Onset of action	Rapid (3–5 minutes)	Rapid (3–5 minutes)[a]	Rapid (3–5 minutes)	Delayed (>15 minutes)
Duration of action	4–6 hours	4–6 hours[b]	>12 hours	>12 hours
Beta-2 adrenoceptor selectivity	Selective	Selective	Selective	Highly selective
Efficacy	Partial agonist	Partial agonist	Full agonist	Partial agonist
Mechanism of action	Direct – salbutamol is hydrophilic and interacts directly with the beta-2 adrenoceptor (fast onset) but does not diffuse into the lipid bilayer (short duration).	Direct –terbutaline is hydrophilic and interacts directly with the beta-2 adrenoceptor (fast onset) but does not diffuse into the lipid bilayer (short duration).	Membrane depot – formoterol is moderately lipophilic, so some drug diffuses into the lipid bilayer (long duration) and at the same time some reaches the aqueous phase and interacts directly with the beta-2 adrenoceptor (fast onset).	Exosite – salmeterol is highly lipophilic, and is retained within the lipid bilayer (long duration) and diffuses only slowly through to reach the beta-2 adrenoceptor (slow onset). Salmeterol hinge theory: the lipophilic side chain of salmeterol binds to the exosite within a hydrophobic part of the beta-2 adrenoceptor and anchors salmeterol to the receptor. This lipophilic side chain of salmeterol acts as a hinge: the 'head' of the salmeterol molecule is involved in repeated engaging and disengaging with the active site of the beta-2 receptor
Clinical role	Reliever/short-term use	Reliever/short-term use	Reliever/maintenance use	Maintenance use

[a] 4–7 hours with bambuterol (prodrug of terbutaline).

[b] 20–24 hours with bambuterol.

Table 10.2 Summary of the dosages and indications of the short-acting beta-2 agonists

Route of administration	Recommended dosage	Indications and comments	UK Proprietary name(s) (manufacturer)
Salbutamol			
Aerosol inhalation	*Adults:* 100–200 mcg (one or two puffs) PRN; for persistent symptoms three or four times daily *Children:* 100 mcg (one puff) PRN, increased to 200 mcg if necessary; for persistent symptoms up to 3–4 times daily **Prophylaxis in EIB** *Adults:* 200 mcg (two puffs) *Children:* 100 mcg (one puff), increased to 200 mcg (two puffs) if necessary	Relief of acute asthma symptoms Prophylaxis in EIB	Salbutamol; non-proprietary (Arrow, Generics, Hillcross, APS) Salamol Easi-Breathe (IVAX) Airomir (IVAX) Ventolin Evohaler (A&H)
Dry powder for inhalation	*Adults:* 200–400 mcg up to three or four times daily *Children:* 200 mcg up to three or four times daily **Prophylaxis in EIB:** 400 mcg (children 200 mcg) Note: bioavailability appears to be lower, so recommended doses for dry-powder inhalers are twice those using a metered dose inhaler	Relief of acute asthma symptoms Prophylaxis in EIB	Pulvinal (Trinity) Cyclocaps (APS) Asmasal Clickhaler (Celltech) Ventodisks (A&H) Ventolin Accuhaler (A&H)
Nebulised solution for inhalation	*Adults and children over 18 months:* 2.5 mg, repeated up to four times daily; increase to 5 mg if necessary (in practice most patients benefit from the 2.5 mg dose) *Children under 18 months (unlicensed):* 1.25–2.5 mg up to four times daily but more frequent administration may be indicated (supplemental oxygen may be required as transient hypoxaemia may occur)	Severe acute asthma Chronic bronchospasm unresponsive to conventional therapy	Salamol Steri-Neb (IVAX) Ventolin Nebules (A&H) Ventolin Respirator solution 5 mg/ml (A&H)

Route of administration	Recommended dosage	Indications and comments	UK Proprietary name(s) (manufacturer)
Oral	**Adults:** 4 mg 3–4 times daily (maximum single dose 8 mg) **Children:** 6–12 years: 2 mg three or four times daily 2–6 years: 1–2 mg three or four times daily Under 2 years (unlicensed): 100 mcg/kg four times daily	Patients with chronic asthma who cannot manage the inhaled route	Salbutamol oral solution and tablets (non-proprietary) Ventmax SR tablets (Trinity) Ventolin syrup (A&H) Volmax tablets (A&H)
Parenteral	**Subcutaneous or intramuscular injection:** 500 mcg, repeated every 4 hours if necessary **Intravenous injection:** 250 mcg, repeated if necessary **Intravenous infusion:** initially 5 mcg/minute, adjusted according to response and heart rate, usually in range 3–20 mcg/minute **Children aged 1 month – 12 years (unlicensed):** 0.1–1 mcg/kg/minute	Chronic asthma (route not usually recommended) Severe asthma	Ventolin (A&H)
Terbutaline			
Aerosol inhalation	**Adults and children:** 250–500 mcg (one or two puffs) PRN; for persistent symptoms up to three or four times daily	Relief of acute asthma symptoms	Bricanyl (AstraZeneca)
Dry powder for inhalation	500 mcg (one inhalation); for persistent symptoms up to three or four times daily	Relief of acute asthma symptoms	Bricanyl Turbohaler (AstraZeneca)
Nebulised solution for inhalation	5–10 mg 2–4 times daily; additional doses may be necessary in severe acute asthma **Children:** up to 3 years: 2 mg 2–4 times daily 3–6 years: 3 mg 2–4 times daily 6–8 years: 4 mg 2–4 times daily over 8 years: 5 mg 2–4 times daily	Severe acute asthma Chronic bronchospasm unresponsive to conventional therapy	Bricanyl Respules Bricanyl Respirator solution 10 mg/ml (all AstraZeneca)

Continued

Table 10.2 Continued

Route of administration	Recommended dosage	Indications and comments	UK Proprietary name(s) (manufacturer)
Oral	Initially 2.5 mg three times daily for 1–2 weeks, then up to 5 mg three times daily *Children:* 75 mcg/kg three times daily 7–15 years: 2.5 mg two or three times daily	Patients with chronic asthma who cannot manage the inhaled route	Bricanyl (tablets and syrup) Bricanyl SA (modified release) (all AstraZeneca)
Parenteral	**Subcutaneous or intramuscular or intravenous injection:** 250–500 mcg up to 4 times daily *Children 2–15 years:* 10 mcg/kg to a maximum of 300 mcg **Continuous intravenous infusion:** solution containing 3–5 mcg/ml, 1.5–5 mcg/minute for 8–10 hours Reduce dosage for children	Chronic asthma (route not usually recommended) Severe asthma	Bricanyl (AstraZeneca)
Bambuterol			
Oral	20 mg once daily at bedtime if patient has previously tolerated beta-2 agonists; other patients, initially 10 mg once daily at bedtime, increased if necessary after 1–2 weeks to 20 mg once daily Not recommended for children	Nocturnal symptoms of asthma (limited role)	Bambec (AstraZeneca)

A&H, Allen & Hanbury; EIB, exercise-induced bronchospasm; mcg, micrograms; PRN, *pro re nata* (as needed).

Table 10.3 Summary of the dosages and indications of the long-acting beta-2 agonists

Route of administration	Recommended dose	Indication and comments	Proprietary name(s) (UK)
Salmeterol			
Inhaled	**Adults**: 50 mcg (two puffs or one blister) twice daily; up to 100 mcg (four puffs or two blisters) twice daily in more severe airways obstruction **Children over 4 years**: 50 mcg (two puffs or one blister) twice daily	Regular long-term treatment of chronic, moderate reversible airways obstruction, including nocturnal asthma and prevention of EIB	Serevent Aerosol, Accuhaler and Diskhaler (Allen & Hanbury)
Formoterol			
Inhaled	**Turbohaler** **Adults (over 18 years)**: 6–12 mcg (4.5–9 mcg[a]) once or twice daily, increased to 24 mcg (18 mcg[a]) twice daily in more severe airways obstruction For short-term symptom relief (but not acute asthma additional doses may be taken to a maximum of 72 mcg (54 mcg[a]) daily (maximum single dose 36 mcg (27 mcg[a]) **Children and adolescents over 6 years**: 12 mcg (9 mcg[a]) once or twice daily (maximum 24 mcg daily) **Prevention of EIB in adults and children over 6 years:** 12 mcg (9 mcg[a]) before exercise **Foradil** 12 mcg twice daily, increased to 24 mcg twice daily in more severe airways obstruction. **Atimos Modulite** **Adults and children over 12 years**: 10.1 mcg twice daily, increased to maximum 20.2 mcg twice daily in more severe airways obstruction	Regular long-term treatment of chronic, moderate reversible airways obstruction, including nocturnal asthma and prevention of EIB	Oxis Turbohaler (AstraZeneca) Foradril Dry power inhaler (Novartis) Atimos Modulite (Trinity-Chiesi)

[a]Each delivered dose (i.e. the dose leaving the mouthpiece) from Oxis Turbohaler contains either 4.5 mcg or 9 mcg formoterol, which is derived from metered doses of 6 mcg and 12 mcg respectively.
EIB, exercise-induced bronchospasm; mcg, micrograms.

between the two drug classes on several inflammatory cells and chemical mediators. Research indicates that beta-2 agonists increase the anti-inflammatory effects of inhaled corticosteroids by enhancing their fundamental action within individual cells. However, the BTS/SIGN asthma management guideline states that there is no difference in efficacy in giving inhaled corticosteroids and long-acting beta agonist in combination or in separate inhalers.[1] There are still no published data showing that a combination inhaler is clinically better than two separate inhalers, but in practice there are positive advantages of using one inhaler if prescribed appropriately. Concordance with an inhaled corticosteroid is a significant problem. The use of combination inhalers can overcome the potential for over-reliance on one controller therapy at the expense of the other, while making it easier for patients to adhere fully to their treatment. One suggested limitation of the fixed-combination inhalers is lack of flexibility, which is potentially important, given the variable airway inflammation inherent to asthma. The two combination treatments currently available offer different management strategies – fixed or adjustable dosing. The salmeterol–fluticasone combination offers a fixed-dose regimen, whereas the formoterol–budesonide combination enables patients to adjust the dose in line with changing symptoms. Cost should also be considered when prescribing combination inhalers, which may be more or less expensive than the separate preparations, depending on the individual dose requirements of each patient. The combined products are summarised in Table 10.4.

Contraindications and special precautions for use

Beta-2 agonists are contraindicated in patients with a history of sensitivity to any of the constituents, and in patients with hypertrophic cardiomyopathy because of their positive inotropic effects. Caution is advised in any patient with myocardial insufficiency or hypokalaemia.

The beta-2 agonists can have hyperglycaemic effects; thus, when used in patients with diabetes, extra blood glucose measurements are recommended initially.

Beta-2 agonists should be administered with caution in patients with thyrotoxicosis.

Asthmatic patients who require therapy with a long-acting beta-2 agonist should also receive regular doses of a corticosteroid. When used without an inhaled corticosteroid, salmeterol has been associated with rare life-threatening attacks of asthma, and high doses of formoterol (e.g. 24 micrograms twice daily) may be associated with an increase in severe

Table 10.4 Summary of the dosages and indications for combination products

Product	Route	Dosage	Indication	Manufacturer
Combivent (ipratropium bromide/salbutamol)	Aerosol inhalation/ nebulised solution for inhalation	Acute severe asthma (unlicensed): inhaled two puffs four times daily nebulised one vial three or four times daily	Not licensed for asthma; ipratropium bromide is only indicated for acute severe asthma In general, patients are best treated with a single-ingredient product so that the dose of each drug can beadjusted	Boehringer Ingelheim
Duovent (one vial contains fenoterol hydrobromide, 1.25 mg, and ipratropium bromide, 500 mcg)	Nebulised solution for inhalation	One vial (4 ml); may be repeated up to a maximum of four vials in 24 hours Not recommended for children under 14 years of age	Acute severe asthma or acute exacerbation of chronic asthma	Boehringer Ingelheim
Seretide Evohaler (salmeterol/fluticasone)	Aerosol inhalation	*Adults and children over 4 years* *Seretide 50*: two puffs twice daily, reduced to two puffs once daily if control is maintained *Adults and children over 12 years* *Seretide 125*: two puffs twice daily *Seretide 250*: two puffs twice daily	Regular long-term treatment of chronic moderate reversible airways obstruction	Allen & Hanbury
Seretide Accuhaler (salmeterol/fluticasone)	Dry powder for inhalation	*Adults and children over 4 years* *Accuhaler 100*: one blister twice daily, reduced to one blister once daily if control is maintained *Adults and children over 12 years* *Accuhaler 250*: one blister twice daily *Accuhaler 500*: one blister twice daily	Regular long-term treatment of chronic moderate reversible airways obstruction	Allen & Hanbury
Symbicort Turbohaler (formoterol/budesonide)	Dry powder for inhalation	**100/6 (fomoterol, 4.5 mcg/budesonide, 80 mcg)** One or two puffs twice daily, increased if necessary to a maximum of four puffs twice daily, reduced to one puff once daily if control is maintained *Adolescents aged 12–17 years*: one or two puffs twice daily, reduced to one puff once daily if control is maintained	Regular long-term treatment of chronic moderate reversible airways obstruction	AstraZeneca

Continued

Table 10.4 Continued

Product	Route	Dosage	Indication	Manufacturer
		Child over 6 years: two puffs twice daily reduced to one puff once daily if control maintained. **200/6 (formoterol, 4.5 mcg/budesonide, 160 mcg)** One or two puffs twice daily, increased if necessary to a maximum of four puffs twice daily, reduced to one puff once daily if control is maintained *Adolescents aged 12–17 years*: one or two puffs twice daily, reduced to one puff once daily if control is maintained Not recommended for children under 12 years **400/12 (formoterol, 9 mcg/budesonide, 320 mcg)** One puff twice daily, increased if necessary to a maximum of two puffs twice daily, reduced to one puff once daily if control is maintained *Adolescents aged 12–17 years*: one puff twice daily, reduced to one puff once daily if control is maintained Not recommended for children under 12 years		

mcg, micrograms.

exacerbations of asthma. Therefore, a long acting beta-2 agonist should be added to existing corticosteroid treatment and not replace it. Patients must be advised to continue taking their corticosteroid after the introduction of a long-acting beta-2 agonist even when symptoms improve.

Adverse effects

Side-effects are dose related and result from stimulation of extrapulmonary beta-2 adrenoceptors. Side-effects are more common with oral or parenteral administration but are rare with inhaled therapy when used within recommended dosages.

The side-effects of long-acting beta-2 agonists are the same as for the short-acting agents and are similarly few when these agents are used via the inhaled route and at recommended dosages.

In the 1960s a number of observations appeared to demonstrate a link between use of high doses of beta-2 agonists and increased asthma mortality, although these findings were not supported by results from larger studies. The risk was greater in patients with more severe and poorly controlled asthma. However, these patients have an increased risk of fatal attacks and are more likely to be using higher doses of beta-2 agonist inhalers and less likely to be using effective anti-inflammatory treatment. Indeed, in the patients who used regular inhaled corticosteroids, there was a significant reduction in risk of death. One study demonstrated that the increased risk of death occurred primarily after usage exceeding two canisters of short-acting beta-2 agonist per month. It is considered good practice that such patients have their medication reviewed to improve asthma control and reduce usage of beta-2 agonists.[1]

The controversy described above increased following the introduction of salmeterol and formoterol. A large multicentre study that examined the safety of salmeterol added to usual care in asthma in 26 355 patients over 12 years of age with asthma who had not previously been treated with a long-acting beta-agonist was terminated when data revealed that the drug may pose a slightly higher risk of respiratory and asthma-related deaths in some patients.[9] Following this study, the Medicines and Healthcare Products Regulatory Agency (MHRA) reminded prescribers that:

- patients given salmeterol or formoterol should always be prescribed an inhaled corticosteroid
- salmeterol or formoterol should not be initiated in patients with acutely deteriorating asthma
- patients should be monitored closely during the first 3 months of treatment.

Skeletal muscle

Muscle tremor and cramps are the most common side-effects and may be troublesome in some elderly patients treated with high doses of beta-2 agonists. The effect is the result of direct stimulation of the skeletal beta-2 adrenoceptors. If possible, the dose of beta-2 agonist should be reduced, or a medication review performed.

Metabolic effects

Hypokalaemia is observed following inhaled or systemic administration of beta-2 agonists. A dose-dependent decrease in the plasma level of potassium ions is observed with increasing doses of these agonists[9] but the change in plasma concentration of potassium ions is minimal at normal therapeutic doses. The hypokalaemia is worsened by co-administration of oral corticosteroids, theophylline or diuretics, and patients should be monitored carefully. Hypokalaemia is mediated by uptake of potassium ions in skeletal muscle. This is potentially serious if the patient is also hypoxic (from poor lung function) and may pre-dispose to cardiac dysrhythmias in acute severe asthma. However, it is important to recognise that tolerance to hypokalaemia is observed with chronic beta-2-agonist therapy.[10]

Increased blood glucose and insulin levels have also been reported and extra blood glucose monitoring is recommended initially.

Respiratory

Beta-2 agonists may reduce arterial oxygen tension (hypoxia) as a con-sequence of ventilation–perfusion mismatching. Such effects may present problems in individuals who have severe hypoxemia before administration of the beta-2 agonist and in young children. These patients may require oxygen supplementation.

Paradoxical bronchospasm occurs on rare occasions and may be caused by the propellant.

Cardiovascular system

Sinus tachycardia, palpitations, prolonged QT interval, vasodilatation and precipitation of cardiac dysrhythmias can occur in susceptible patients. These events may be caused by a direct effect of beta-2 agonists on atrial beta-2 adrenoceptors, combined with a reflex cardiac stimulation resulting from the increase in peripheral vasodilatation mediated via beta-2 adrenoceptors.

Central nervous system

Headache, restlessness, tension, dizziness, nervousness and insomnia may occur.

Tolerance

Tolerance to side-effects may develop with continuous treatment because of down-regulation of beta-2 adrenoceptors (i.e. the number of beta adrenoceptors on cells decreases). Tolerance to the bronchodilator effects may occur in some people, although the duration of action tends to be affected more than the peak effect attained. Thus, short-acting beta-2 agonists, when used regularly, will maintain effectiveness for a diminished period but the peak bronchodilator effect is better preserved and they continue to perform well as reliever medication.

Tolerance can also mean a reduction in the bronchoprotective effect against challenge with bronchoconstrictor stimuli (i.e. taking a beta-2 agonist before being exposed to methacholine, histamine, AMP, allergen, exercise or cold air). The bronchoprotection is not completely lost but is reduced from its initial level.

The adverse effects of the beta-2 agonist are summarised in the Adverse Effects Focus on page 166.

Drug interactions

The beta-2 agonists do not have significant interactions with any drugs other than beta-blockers. Co-administration of beta-2 agonists with the following drugs merits caution.

- The effects of beta-2 agonists are inhibited by beta-blockers, especially those without beta-1-receptor selectivity (i.e. the non-selective beta-blockers).
- Xanthine derivatives, steroids and diuretics may potentiate the possible hypokalaemic effect of beta-2 agonists.
- Monoamine oxidase inhibitors may cause hypertensive reactions.

Bambuterol may interact with suxamethonium (succinylcholine). A prolongation of the muscle-relaxing effect of suxamethonium of up to twofold has been observed in some patients after taking bambuterol,

Adverse effects of beta-2 agonists

Site	Adverse effect	Mechanism
Skeletal muscle	Muscle tremor	Stimulation of beta-2 adrenoceptors in skeletal muscle
Cardiovascular system	Tachycardia and palpitations	Reflex cardiac stimulation secondary to vasodilatation, direct stimulation of atrial beta-2 adrenoceptors and possibly also stimulation of myocardial beta-1 adrenoceptors at higher doses
Metabolic effects (seen only after large systemic doses)	Increase in free fatty acids, insulin, glucose and lactate concentrations. Hypokalaemia	Beta-2-adrenoceptor-mediated stimulation of potassium entry into skeletal muscle. Hypokalaemia may be serious in the presence of hypoxia, as in acute asthma, when there may be a predisposition to cardiac dysrhythmias
Respiratory	Increased ventilation–perfusion mismatching	Pulmonary vasodilatation in blood vessels previously constricted by hypoxia, resulting in shunting of blood to poorly ventilated areas and a fall in arterial oxygen tension; in practice, the change in partial pressure of oxygen is very small (<5 mmHg)
Central nervous system	Headache, restlessness, tension, dizziness, nervousness, insomnia	Stimulation of beta-2 adrenoceptors

20 mg, on the evening before surgery. The interaction is dose dependent and arises because plasma cholinesterase, which inactivates suxamethonium, is partly, but fully reversibly, inhibited by bambuterol. In extreme situations, the interaction may result in a prolonged apnoea time, which may be of clinical importance.

Preparations

Tables 10.2 and 10.3 summarise the preparations of short-acting and long-acting beta-2 blockers, respectively. Table 10.4 summarises the combination products that contain beta-2 agonists.

References

1. British Thoracic Society/Scottish Intercollegiate Guidelines Network. British Guideline on the Management of Asthma. *Thorax* 2003; 58 (Suppl I): S1–S94.
2. Anderson GP, Linden A, Rabe KF. Why are long-acting beta-adrenoceptor agonists long-acting? *Eur Respir J* 1994; 7: 569–578.
3. Johnson M. Beta-2-adrenoceptors: mechanisms of action of beta-2 agonists. *Paediatr Respir Rev* 2001; 2: 57–62.
4. Devalia JL, Sapsford RJ, Rusznak C, *et al*. The effects of salmeterol and salbutamol on ciliary beat frequency of cultured human bronchial epithelial cells, in vitro. *Pulm Pharmacol* 1992; 5: 257–263.
5. Dowling RB, Johnson M, Cole PJ, *et al*. Effect of salmeterol on *Haemophilus influenzae* infection of respiratory mucosa *in vitro*. *Eur Respir J* 1998; 11: 86–90.
6. Tattersfield AE, Lofdhal CG, Postma DS, *et al*. Comparison of formoterol and terbutaline for as-needed treatment of asthma; a randomised trial. *Lancet* 2001; 357: 257–261.
7. Crompton GK, Ayres JG, Basran G, *et al*. Comparison of oral bambuterol and inhaled salmeterol in patients with symptomatic asthma and using inhaled corticosteroids. *Am J Respir Crit Care Med* 1999; 159: 824–828.
8. Wallaert B, Brun P, Ostinelli J, *et al*. A comparison of two long-acting beta-agonists, oral bambuterol and inhaled salmeterol, in the treatment of moderate to severe asthmatic patients with nocturnal symptoms. The French Bambuterol Study Group. *Respir Med* 1999; 93: 33–38.
9. Harold S, Nelson MD, Scott T, *et al*. The Salmeterol Multicentre Asthma Research Trial: A comparison of usual pharmacotherapy for asthma or usual pharmacotherapy plus salmeterol. *Chest* 2006; 129: 15–26.
10. Wong CS, Pavord ID, Williams J, *et al*. Bronchodilator, cardiovascular and hypokalaemic effects of fenoterol, salbutamol and terbutaline in asthma. *Lancet* 1990; 336: 1396–1399.
11. Lipworth BJ, Struthers AD, McDevitt DG. Tachyphylaxis to systemic but not to airway responses during prolonged therapy with high dose inhaled salbutamol in asthmatics. *Am Rev Respir Dis* 1989; 140: 586–592.

11

Anticholinergics

Indications

Atropine, a naturally occurring compound from the plant *Atropa belladonna* (Deadly Nightshade), was the first anticholinergic to be used in the treatment of asthma. However, the side-effects were too troublesome, and less-soluble quaternary compounds such as ipratropium bromide were introduced (Figure 11.1).

Responsiveness to anticholinergics varies widely among asthmatic patients: some patients respond very little whereas others respond almost as well to these drugs as to beta-2 agonists. It is difficult to identify subgroups of patients who are most likely to respond. Studies reported in the 1980s suggested that individuals with intrinsic asthma and those with longer duration of asthma may respond better than individuals with extrinsic or recent-onset asthma.[1,2] However, the definitions of asthma versus chronic obstructive pulmonary disease (COPD) were less clearly defined at that time, so this suggestion needs to be interpreted with care. Anticholinergics are potent bronchodilators in patients with COPD.[3] Today, the inhaled anticholinergics are rarely used to treat asthma, as they are less potent bronchodilators than the beta-2 agonists. The most recent British Thoracic Society/Scottish Intercollegiate Network (BTS/SIGN) asthma management guideline[4] does not include anticholinergics in the management of stable asthma but it does recommend the addition of short-acting anticholinergics in acute asthma if the patient has not responded to short-acting beta-2 agonists.

In some, but not all, patients with acute exacerbations of asthma, ipratropium bromide has been shown to have additive effects with inhaled short-acting beta-2 agonists. In a large study (n = 199), Rebuck and colleagues gave patients a combination of ipratropium bromide 500 micrograms with fenoterol 1.25 mg via nebuliser.[5] The combination resulted in significantly more bronchodilation over the first 90 minutes of treatment than either agent alone. It is therefore appropriate to recommend use of ipratropium bromide in combination with

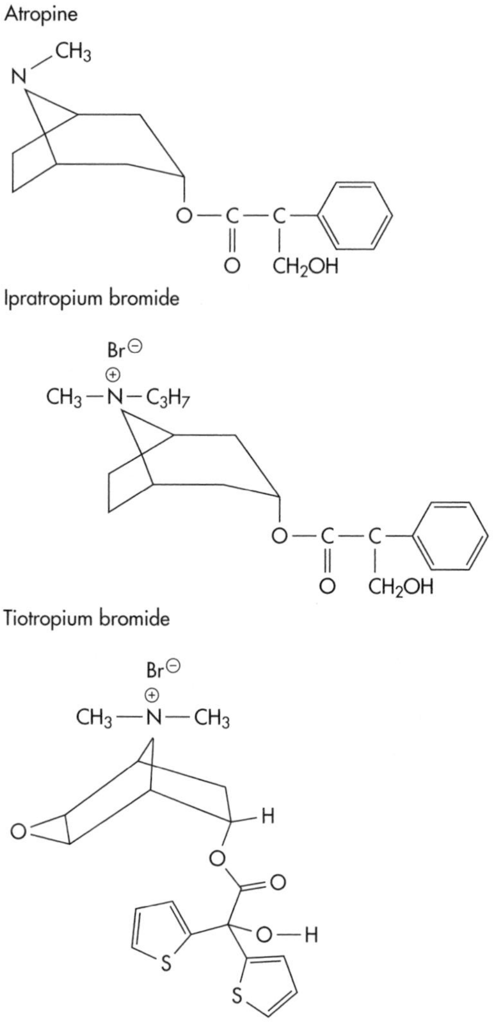

Atropine

Ipratropium bromide

Tiotropium bromide

Figure 11.1 Chemical structures of atropine, ipratropium bromide and tiotropium bromide.

a beta-2 agonist in acute severe asthma, especially in the early hours of treatment and particularly in patients with more severe airflow obstruction. The BTS/SIGN British asthma guideline[4] recommends the addition of short-acting anticholinergics in acute asthma if the patient has not responded to short-acting beta-2 agonists. The optimal duration of combination therapy in this setting is between 12 and 36 hours.[6] Anticholinergic treatment is not necessary and may not be beneficial in milder exacerbations of asthma or after stabilisation.

Mechanism of action

The anticholinergics are competitive antagonists at the muscarinic acetylcholine receptor. There are three main muscarinic receptors in the human airway: M1, M2 and M3 (Figure 11.2).[7] M1 receptors are localised within the parasympathetic ganglia and their blockade reduces reflex bronchoconstriction. M2 receptors are located at cholinergic nerve terminals and act as autoreceptors, inhibiting the release of acetylcholine. Bronchoconstriction and mucus secretion are stimulated via M3 receptors. Ipratropium bromide has activity against M1, M2 and M3 receptors. By blocking these receptors, ipratropium bromide inhibits cholinergic reflex bronchoconstriction and reduces vagal cholinergic tone, leading to bronchodilation, and decreases mucus secretion.

Tiotropium bromide is a relatively new anticholinergic licensed for the treatment of COPD, but not asthma. It is a selective antagonist of both the M1 and M3 receptor subtypes that mediate bronchoconstriction and has a long duration of action (24 hours).[8-10]

Pharmacological properties

Ipratropium bromide and tiotropium bromide are quaternary compounds, which are poorly absorbed from the gastrointestinal tract. These agents are fully anticholinergic at the site of deposition: they dilate the pupil if delivered directly to the eye and dilate the bronchi when inhaled. Following inhalation, uptake into the plasma is minimal. The peak blood concentration occurs within 3 hours of inhalation. Excretion is via the kidneys.

The onset of bronchodilation following inhalation of ipratropium bromide is relatively slow compared with that seen with the beta-2 agonists, the peak effect occurring after 30–90 minutes. The bronchodilation is sustained for 6–8 hours. Ipratropium bromide should be administered three or four times a day.

Dosage

Ipratropium bromide

As mentioned above, the addition of an anticholinergic in the routine management of a patient with stable asthma is generally of no value[11] but the addition of a short-acting anticholinergic may be useful in the management of acute asthma if the patient has not responded to short-acting beta-2 agonists.

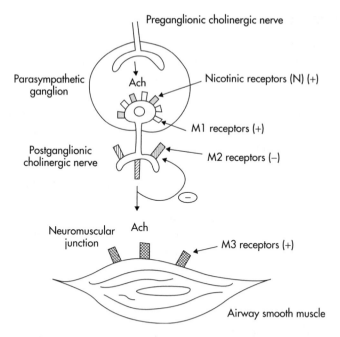

Figure 11.2 Muscarinic receptor subtypes. (From: Hansel T and Barnes P. *The Encylopedia of Visual Medicine Series. An Atlas of COPD.* London, Parthenon Publishing Group, 2004; Figure 5.15. Reproduced with permission of the Taylor and Francis Group.)

Ipratropium bromide is available as a nebulised solution for inhalation, in a metered-dose inhaler, in an autohaler and as dry powder for inhalation. Generally the nebuliser route is prescribed for acute severe or life-threatening asthma and for those with a poor initial response to beta-2-agonist therapy. The optimal dose of ipratroprium bromide via a nebuliser in adults is 500 micrograms up to four times daily; the total recommended daily dose of 2 mg should not be exceeded during either acute or maintenance treatment. The recommended dose in children is 250 micrograms up to a total daily dose of 1 mg for children aged 6–12 years and 125–250 micrograms for children up to 5 years of age, up to a total of 1 mg daily. The time interval between doses can be determined by the prescriber but ipratropium bromide should not be administered more frequently than 6 hourly to children under 5 years of age.

The metered-dose inhaler is licensed for the relief of acute asthma symptoms (reversible airway obstruction). The recommended dosage for adults is 20–40 micrograms (one or two puffs) three or four times daily although some patients may need up to 80 micrograms at a time to obtain maximum benefit during early treatment. A dose of 20 micrograms three times daily is recommended for children up to 6 years, and 20–40 micrograms three times daily for children aged 6–12 years. There is limited experience of the use of ipratropium dry powder inhaler in children, therefore the product is not recommended for use in children under 12 years. In adults the licensed dose is 40 micrograms three or four times daily which may be doubled in less responsive patients.

Combination bronchodilator preparations

Combivent (Boehringer Ingelheim) contains ipratropium bromide and salbutamol (a short-acting beta-2 agonist). Combivent is available as both a metered-dose inhaler and a nebuliser solution. Combivent is not licensed for the treatment of asthma but it is commonly prescribed off license for acute asthma when both drugs are indicated.

Duovent contains ipratropium bromide 500 micrograms and fenoterol (short-acting beta-2 agonist) 1.25 mg. It is only available as a nebuliser solution in the UK and is licensed for acute severe asthma or acute exacerbation of chronic asthma at a dose of one vial (4 ml), which can be repeated up to a maximum of four vials in a 24 hour period. Duovent is not recommended in children under 14 years of age.

Contraindications

Anticholinergic preparations should not be taken by patients with known hypersensitivity to atropine or its derivatives, or to any other component of the product.

Adverse effects

Inhaled delivery with virtually no systemic absorption means that adverse effects are uncommon. In normal clinical practice, the only side-effects that the patient might experience with ipratropium bromide are dryness of the mouth and a brief coughing spell, which has been reported to occur in 5% of patients[12] (see Adverse Effects Focus, page 174).

Anticholinergics can cause eye pain, blurred vision, visual halos and conjunctival and corneal congestion (redness). In patients susceptible to glaucoma, care should be taken to avoid contact of the drug with the eyes, particularly when ipratropium bromide is given by nebuliser or in combination with a beta-2 agonist. To avoid acute-angle-closure glaucoma, it is recommended that ipratropium is nebulised with a mouthpiece in preference to a nebuliser mask.

Anticholinergic agents are unlikely to increase hypoxaemia,[13] as the beta-2 agonists do, an important consideration in exacerbations of

ADVERSE EFFECTS FOCUS

Adverse effects of anticholinergics	
Local	**Systemic**
• Dry mouth	• Headache
• Cough	• Nervousness and irritation
• Sore throat	• Dizziness
• Bitter metallic taste	• Supraventricular tachycardia
• Upper respiratory tract infection	• Atrial fibrillation
• Nausea	• Urinary difficulty
• Acute-angle-closure glaucoma, eye pain, blurred vision, visual halos, conjunctival and corneal congestion (redness)	• Urinary retention
	• Constipation
• Paradoxical (inhalation) bronchoconstriction is usually caused by additives in the nebuliser solution	

asthma and COPD. Mucociliary clearance is unaffected by anticholinergics, although mucus secretion may be decreased.

Drug interactions

No drug interactions have been reported during trials with ipratropium bromide.

Preparations

Ipratropium bromide is the most widely used anticholinergic in the UK. It is available as a metered-dose inhaler and a nebulised preparation.
The following preparations are available:

- Atrovent aerosol for inhalation (Boehringer Ingelheim)
- Atrovent nebuliser solution (Boehringer Ingelheim)
- Atrovent dry powder (Aerocaps) for inhalation (Boehringer Ingelheim)
- Respontin nebuliser solution (Allen & Hanbury)
- Ipratropium Steri-Neb (IVAX)
- Ipratropium bromide nebuliser solution (Galen, Generics)

- Combivent (ipratropium bromide and salbutamol) aerosol for inhalation and nebuliser solution (Boehringer Ingelheim)
- Duovent (ipratropium bromide and fenoterol hydrochloride) nebuliser solution (Boehringer Ingelheim).

References

1. Ullah MI, Newman GB, Saunders KB. Influence of age on response to ipratropium and salbutamol in asthma. *Thorax* 1981; 36: 523–529.
2. Jolobe OM. Asthma versus non-specific reversible airflow obstruction: clinical features and responsiveness to anticholinergic drugs. *Respiration* 1984; 45: 237–242.
3. Braun SR, Levy SF. Comparison of ipratropium bromide and albuterol in chronic obstructive pulmonary disease: a three-centre study. *Am J Med* 2002; 91 (Suppl 4A): 28S–32S.
4. British Thoracic Society/Scottish Intercollegiate Guidelines Network. British Guideline on the Management of Asthma. *Thorax* 2003; 58 (Suppl I): S1–S94.
5. Rebuck AS, Chapman KR, Abbound R, *et al.* Nebulised anticholinergic and sympathomimetic treatment of asthma and chronic obstructive airways disease in the emergency room. *Am J Med* 1987; 82: 59–64.
6. Brophy C, Ahmed B, Bayston S, *et al.* How long should Atrovent be given in acute asthma? *Thorax* 1998; 53: 363–367.
7. Barnes PJ. Muscarinic receptor subtypes in airways. *Life Sci* 1993; 52: 521–528.
8. Hansel TT, Barnes PJ. Tiotropium: a novel once-daily anticholinergic bronchodilator for the treatment of COPD. *Drugs Today* 2002; 38: 585–600.
9. Barnes PJ. Tiotropium bromide. *Expert Opin Investig Drugs* 2001; 10: 733–740.
10. Hvizdos KM, Goa KL. Tiotropium bromide. *Drugs* 2002; 62: 1195–1203.
11. Pharmacological management of asthma. Evidence table 4.11c: add-on drugs for inhaled steroids: anticholinergics. Edinburgh: SIGN; 2002. Available from http: //www.sign.ac.uk/guidelines/published/support/guideline63/index.html
12. Tashkin DP, Ashutosh K, Bleecker ER, *et al.* Comparison of the anticholinergic bronchodilator ipratropium bromide with metaproterenol in chronic obstructive pulmonary disease. A 90 day multi-centre study. *Am J Med* 1986; 81(5A): 81–90.
13. Gross NJ, Bankwala Z. Effects of an anticholinergic bronchodilator on arterial blood gases of hypoxaemic patients with chronic obstructive pulmonary disease. Comparison with a beta-adrenergic agent. *Am Rev Respir Dis* 1987; 136: 1091–1094.

12

Corticosteroids

Indications

The most important aspect of managing chronic asthma is controlling the inflammatory component of the disease. If the inflammation is well controlled, there will be fewer exacerbations and these will be less serious. Corticosteroids are the most effective therapy currently available for asthma. They were introduced for the treatment of asthma shortly after their discovery in the 1950s. For routine long-term, management of asthma, corticosteroids are given by inhalation, which reduces the risk of side-effects quite considerably compared with oral administration. Inhaled corticosteroids (ICSs) are now recommended as first-line therapy for all but the mildest asthma, although the exact threshold for introduction of an ICS has yet to be established. Two recent studies have shown benefit from regular use of an ICS in patients with mild asthma.[1,2] The British Thoracic Society/Scottish Intercollegiate Guidelines Network (BTS/SIGN) asthma management guideline recommends that an ICS is are considered for patients with any of the following:[3]

- exacerbations of asthma in the last 2 years
- use of inhaled beta-2 agonists three times a week or more
- symptoms three times a week or more, or waking one night a week or more because of asthma.

Oral dosing may be necessary during severe exacerbations or in very severe asthma, however.

The most widely used ICSs are beclometasone diproprionate, budesonide and fluticasone propionate. Mometasone and ciclesonide were introduced more recently, both formulated in an inhaler for the treatment of asthma. The structures of the ICSs are shown in Figure 12.1.

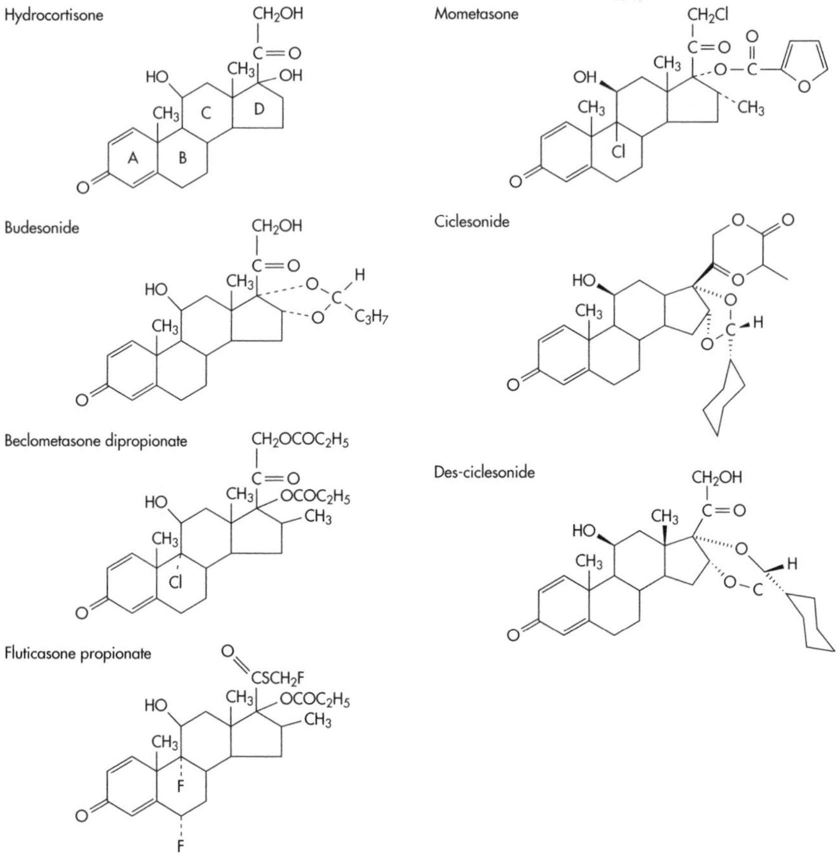

Figure 12.1 Chemical structures of hydrocortisone, budesonide, beclometasone, ciclesonide, fluticasone and mometasone. Hydrocortisone contains the characteristic steroid nucleus, consisting of three six-carbon rings (ABC), and a single five-carbon ring (D). Hydrocortisone is the major glucocorticoid produced by the adrenal cortex. Beclometasone dipropionate, budesonide, ciclesonide, fluticasone and mometasone are synthetic analogs of hydrocortisone. Des-ciclesonide is the active metabolite of ciclesonide.

Mechanism of action[4]

Molecular mechanisms

Corticosteroids provide highly effective anti-inflammatory therapy in asthma. The mechanism of action is highly complex. They act in a relatively non-specific manner by inhibiting cytokine expression, transcription factors and a variety of inflammatory cells involved in the disease process.

When corticosteroids are inhaled, they enter the target cells in the lung and bind to a single class of glucocorticoid receptors localised in the cytoplasm of target cells. Following steroid binding, the receptor is activated. The steroid–receptor complex dimerises and translocates to the nucleus, where it binds to specific DNA sequences, usually termed glucocorticoid response elements (GRE). This interaction changes the rate of transcription of a wide range of inflammatory mediators (e.g cytokines, histamine, leukotrienes), resulting in either induction or repression of the gene. It usually increases transcription, resulting in increased protein synthesis. However, most of the anti-inflammatory effects of corticosteroids are thought to be mediated by the repression of transcription factors.[5] The endocrine and metabolic effects of corticosteroids are thought to be mediated via GRE binding.

Several other activated transcription factors bind directly to the glucocorticoid receptors. This protein–protein interaction may regulate the expression of genes that code for inflammatory proteins, such as cytokines, inflammatory enzymes, adhesion molecules and inflammatory receptors. This could be an important determinant of corticosteroid responsiveness and is a key mechanism whereby corticosteroids switch off inflammatory genes.

Overall corticosteroids act by:

- increasing the synthesis of anti-inflammatory proteins, such as lipocortin-1 which has an inhibitory effect on phospholipase A2
- reducing the number and activity of mucosal mast cells, eosinophils and neutrophils
- reducing the secretion of chemokines and pro-inflammatory cytokines from alveolar macrophages
- increasing the secretion of interleukin-10
- preventing and reversing the increased vascular permeability and therefore reducing airway oedema
- reducing mucus secretion in the mucous membranes
- up-regulating beta-adrenoceptor populations and sensitivity (this may prevent down-regulation of beta-2 adrenoceptors in response to prolonged treatment with beta-2 agonists)[6]
- suppressing the late-phase inflammatory response (see Chapter 2) (ICSs have no effect on the early response to allergen, reflecting their lack of effect on mediator release from mast cells)
- inhibiting the increase in airway hyperresponsiveness (this effect may take several weeks or months to develop; long-term treatment with ICSs reduces responsiveness to histamine, cholinergic agonists, allergens,

exercise, fog, cold air, bradykinin, adenosine and irritants such as sulphur and metabisulfite).

It is important to recognise that corticosteroids suppress inflammation in the airways but do not cure the underlying disease. When corticosteroids are withdrawn, the pre-treatment degree of airway hyper-responsiveness will return, although in mild asthma this may take several months.

Clinical mechanisms

ICSs are highly effective in controlling asthma symptoms of various severity in patients of all ages. They improve the quality of life of many patients, allowing them to lead normal lives. They also improve patients' lung function, reduce the frequency of exacerbations and may prevent irreversible airway changes (see Management Focus, below).

Pharmacokinetics

All ICSs exert their pharmacological effects through the same mechanism. Variations in efficacy and adverse effects seen with the different preparations are a result of differences in their pharmacokinetic profiles. The pharmacokinetics of an ICS are important in determining the lung deposition of the drug and the amount of the drug that reaches the systemic circulation and thus causes adverse effects.[7] The ideal ICS is one that has a high topical potency acting locally in the airway mucosa, a low systemic bioavailability of the swallowed portion of the drug, minimal absorption from the airways and alveolar surface into the systemic circulation and rapid clearance of any corticosteroid that does reach the systemic circulation. The Management Focus on page 181

MANAGEMENT FOCUS

Effects of inhaled corticosteroids in asthma

- Control symptoms
- Prevent/reduce exacerbations
- Improve lung function
- Prevent irreversible airway changes (remodelling)
- Improve quality of life
- Reduce mortality (probably)

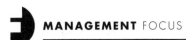 **MANAGEMENT** FOCUS

Ideal pharmacokinetics and pharmacodynamic properties of an inhaled corticosteroid for the long-term treatment of asthma

---

Ideal pharmacokinetic properties

- Low oral bioavailability
- Low systemic bioavailability
- High pulmonary bioavailability
- High glucocorticoid receptor binding affinity
- High plasma protein binding
- Pro-drug structure
- Large volume of distribution
- High lipid conjugation
- High lipophilicity
- Rapid systemic clearance

Ideal pharmacodynamic properties

- High pulmonary deposition
- Prolonged residence time
- Small particle size

---

summarises the desirable pharmacodynamic and pharmacokinetic properties of an ideal ICS for the long-term management of asthma.

Deposition and bioavailability

Systemic bioavailability is the amount of the drug that becomes systemically available after absorption from the lung, gastrointestinal absorption and first-pass metabolism of the swallowed fraction of the dose. Oral bioavailability is low for most of the more recently developed ICSs; most of the systemically available corticosteroid therefore comes from the inhaled fraction that enters the systemic circulation after absorption from the lung. As systemically available corticosteroid is responsible for the observed systemic adverse effects, it is desirable to have the lowest systemic bioavailability possible. For optimum efficacy and safety, high pulmonary bioavailability coupled with low oral bioavailability is desirable.

After inhalation, a proportion of the inhaled dose is deposited on the oropharynx. It is then swallowed and is available for absorption via the gastrointestinal tract into the systemic circulation (see Figure 12.2).

The fraction that is deposited differs between the different ICSs and is markedly reduced by the use of a large-volume spacer device. Rinsing the mouth and discarding the rinse also reduces systemic absorption and all patients should be encouraged to do this. The absorbed fraction may be metabolised by the liver (first-pass metabolism), reducing the amount that reaches the systemic circulation. Fluticasone, ciclesonide and mometasone undergo almost complete first-pass metabolism and therefore have negligible oral bioavailability (<1%) and may therefore cause fewer systemic adverse effects, although absorption of the drug from the airway must be considered. In comparison, beclometasone monopropionate has an oral bioavailability of 26% and budesonide 11%.[8]

The inhaled portion of an ICS that is not deposited on the oropharynx is deposited in the airway, where it exerts its pharmacological action and becomes available for absorption into the systemic circulation. The percentage deposited in the airway varies between the different drugs and inhaler devices. MDIs are relatively inefficient since typically only 10–20% of the actuated drug is deposited in the lungs; 70–80% is swallowed and up to 10% exhaled. Many factors affect

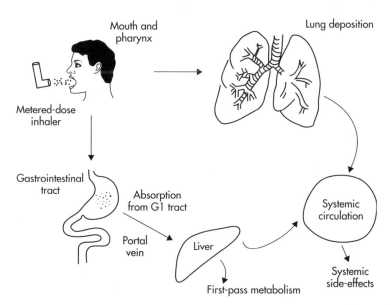

Figure 12.2 Absorption of inhaled corticosteroids. The potential systemic effects of inhaled corticosteroids depend on the amount of inhaled corticosteroid absorbed through the airways and the amount absorbed from the gastrointestinal tract that is not metabolised on first pass through the liver.

deposition of the drug in the lung (see Chapter 7). The aim is to produce an inhaler that enables deposition of a high proportion of the drug in the lung so that more of the drug can reach its target. For example, deposition of ICS particles is increased by one of the hydrofluoroalkane formulations of beclometasone dipropionate (QVAR) which has a finer particle size. The newly licensed ciclesonide inhaler has been designed to reduce the fraction of active corticosteroid absorbed via the respiratory tract by improving the retention of the drug within the airway. Lung deposition with ciclesonide is approximately 52%.

Receptor affinity and local retention

The potency of ICSs can be estimated by measuring their binding affinity for corticosteroid receptors. The *in vitro* binding affinities of the currently available corticosteroids are shown in Table 12.1. However, it is important to appreciate that the effectiveness of corticosteroids depends on more complex interactions than basic receptor binding alone. The corticosteroid must be retained in the target tissue in sufficient concentrations for a sufficient time span if it is to exert any therapeutic effect. It should also diffuse readily through cell membranes, with little or no metabolic inactivation, in order to reach the glucocorticoid receptor. The residence time of an ICS in the airways depends on the stability of the drug and its lipid solubility (lipophilicity).

The binding affinity of beclometasone appears unfavourable when compared with that of other ICSs but beclometasone is further activated in the lung by metabolism to 17-beclometasone monopropionate. This metabolite has a relative affinity for glucocorticoid receptors that is 20 higher than that of beclometasone (Table 12.1).

Budesonide has a slightly lower binding affinity than other ICSs but, again, this may be misleading. Budesonide undergoes esterification in the lung to form an inactive intracellular lipid conjugate of budesonide which acts as a local depot for its slow release. As the intracellular concentration of budesonide decreases, the esterified budesonide is hydrolysed and active budesonide is released from the depot. Budesonide is thus retained in airway tissue to a greater extent and this prolonged exposure to the glucocorticoid receptors in the airways increases its anti-inflammatory effects.

Ciclesonide is inhaled as an inactive parent compound that is converted to its active form in the airways. Ciclesonide itself has a low binding affinity for the glucocorticoid receptor, but in the airways it is hydrolysed to its active metabolite, des-ciclesonide, which has a high affinity for the glucocorticoid receptor. Des-ciclesonide forms a fatty-acid-ester conjugate in the lung, which acts as a pool for its slow release, increasing the exposure time with the glucocorticoid receptors. This provides the rationale behind the once-daily prescribing of ciclesonide.

Fluticasone is highly lipophilic, which promotes its entry into cells, allows rapid binding to glucocorticoid receptors and aids retention in the lung tissue. Fluticasone has a high affinity for lung glucocorticoid receptors, which is three-fold higher than that of budesonide.

Mometasone possesses a high binding affinity for the glucocorticoid receptor – higher than that of fluticasone and budesonide.

Protein binding

Protein-bound corticosteroids cannot exert pharmacological effects, as they are unable to bind to the glucocorticoid receptor. Only free, unbound drug is capable of interacting with the receptor. High protein binding is advantageous because this results in low systemic concentrations of unbound drug, which improve the risk–benefit ratio by lowering the risk for systemic adverse effects.

Distribution and elimination

Tissue distribution (expressed as volume of distribution) shows a marked variation among the various ICSs and correlates strongly with lipophilicity. Fluticasone appears to be the most widely distributed of the currently available corticosteroids, with a volume of distribution 3–5 times higher than that of most of the other ICSs. In general for an ICS, a greater volume of distribution indicates a greater tissue distribution in the lung and thus greater potential for glucocorticoid receptor binding.

ICSs are primarily eliminated by oxidative liver metabolism. Clearance is similar for most of the ICSs. Rapid clearance of drug absorbed systemically is desirable, in order to minimise adverse effects resulting from systemic exposure.

The pharmacokinetic properties of the corticosteroids most commonly used in asthma are shown in Table 12.1.

Dose–response relationships

The dose–response curve for the clinical anti-asthmatic efficacy of the ICSs is relatively flat and tends to plateau at daily doses above 800 micrograms beclometasone or budesonide in adults and 400 micrograms

Table 12.1 Pharmacodynamic and pharmacokinetic properties of inhaled corticosteroids commonly used in the treatment of asthma

	Receptor binding affinity[a]	Oral broavailability	Plasma protein binding	Fatty acid conjugation	Steady-state volume of distribution (L)	Elimination half-life (hours)	Clearance (L/hour)
Beclometasone diproprionate	0.5	15–20%	87%	No	20	0.5	150
17-Beclometasone monopropionate	13.45	26%	ND	No	424	2.7	120
Budesonide	9.4	11%	88%	Yes	183–301	2.8	84
Ciclesonide	0.12	<1%	99%	No	207	0.36	152
Des-ciclesonide[b]	12.0	<1%	99%	Yes	897–1310	3.4	228
Fluticasone	22.0	<1%	90%	No	318–859	7–8	66–90
Mometasone furoate	23.0	<1%	89–99%	No	152	5.8	54

[a] A low value indicates a poor affinity of the corticosteroid for the glucocorticoid receptor; [b] active metabolite of ciclesonide.
ND, not determined.

in children with mild-to-moderate asthma (see Figure 12.3). Systemic adverse effects may occur above this threshold. However, there is considerable variation between patients in the dose–response relationship, both in the airways and systemically. Most benefits in patients with asthma have been demonstrated at lower doses of ICSs. The dose–response effect has largely been demonstrated by measuring traditional lung function parameters; further studies are required to determine dose–response effects in prevention of asthma exacerbations, airway hyperresponsiveness and sputum eosinophilia.

Time course of response

Generally, the cellular and biochemical effects mediated by oral corticosteroids are immediate, but varying amounts of time are required to produce clinical response. In acute severe asthma, 4–12 hours may be required before any clinical response is noted.

The response to an ICS is not immediate. For most patients, symptoms improve in the first 1–2 weeks of therapy and reach maximum improvement in 4–8 weeks. Improvements in bronchial hyperresponsiveness may take up to 3 months and may continue to show improvement over 12 months of therapy.

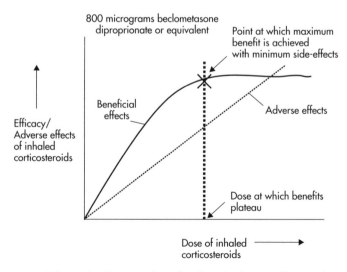

Figure 12.3 Relationship between beneficial and adverse effects with increasing doses of inhaled corticosteroids. (From: Chung F. Current approaches to asthma management. *Prescriber* 5 March 2003; Reproduced with permission from Wiley Interface Ltd.)

Dosage

Several ICSs can be prescribed in the UK for asthma. It has often proved difficult to establish true differences in clinical efficacy between the different preparations. Various studies have shown differences in the efficacy and safety but these have not been consistent. Budesonide and beclometasone appear to have comparable anti-asthma effects at equal doses in adults and children. Both mometasone and fluticasone appear to be approximately twice as potent as beclometasone-CFC and are given at half the dose. The dose of HFA-based beclometasone (QVAR) is approximately half that of the CFC-based beclometasone preparations.[3] The therapeutic relativity of ciclesonide to other ICSs is not yet established conclusively.

An ICS should be started at a dose that reflects the severity of the patient's asthma. In mild-to-moderate asthma, starting at a high dose of ICS and stepping down confers no benefit.[9] An appropriate starting dose would be beclometasone (or equivalent) 400 micrograms daily in adults and 200 micrograms daily in children aged 5 years and over. Higher doses may be required in children under 5 years if there are problems in achieving consistent drug delivery.[3] The dose of ICS should be titrated to the lowest dose at which effective control of asthma is maintained. Previous advice from the BTS asthma management guideline was to increase the dose of ICS up to at least 2000 micrograms beclometasone or equivalent if asthma was not controlled by standard doses. However, it is now apparent that the dose–response effect of the ICSs is relatively flat and there is little improvement in lung function above beclometasone, 800 micrograms daily. It is therefore recommended to add in another controller agent[10–12] (covered in more detail in Chapter 3).

ICSs must be taken regularly. When they are discontinued there is usually a gradual increase in symptoms back to pre-treatment values.

Many studies have shown that twice-daily administration of ICSs gives comparable control to administration four times daily. Furthermore, in patients who require less than 400 micrograms daily, once-daily dosing appears to be as effective as twice-daily dosing.[13] Once-daily dosing at the same total daily dose can be considered (within product licence) if good control is established.

Intravenous hydrocortisone can be given in acute severe asthma. The recommended dose is 400 mg daily (100 mg every 6 hours) intravenously. Oral prednisolone has a similar effect to intravenous hydrocortisone and is the preferred treatment unless there are contraindications to oral therapy. Oral prednisolone should be prescribed in doses of 40–50 mg daily. For convenience, steroid tablets may be given as 2 × 25 mg tablets daily rather than 8–12 × 5 mg tablets. The oral corticosteroid should be continued at this dose for at least 5 days or until recovery. Steroid tablets can be stopped abruptly after recovery from the acute exacerbation and the dosage does not need tapering, provided the patient receives an ICS (apart from patients on maintenance steroid treatment or rare instances where steroids are required for 3 weeks or more).[14]

Contraindications

There are no specific contraindications for inhaled therapy but caution is required in patients with pulmonary tuberculosis or fungal or viral respiratory infections.

Except where their use may be life-saving, oral corticosteroids must be used with great caution in patients with the following conditions: peptic ulcer, osteoporosis, infections (including tuberculosis), hypertension, congestive heart failure, liver failure, renal insufficiency, diabetes mellitus or a family history of diabetes, epilepsy and/or seizure disorders, previous steroid myopathy, myasthenia gravis treated with anticholinesterase therapy, thromboembolic disorders and psychological disturbances.

Adverse effects

Adverse effects can be divided into local and systemic effects. Local adverse effects result from the deposition of the corticosteroid from the inhaler into the oropharyngeal spaces; systemic effects arise from corticosteroid absorbed into the systemic circulation from the airways and lungs, from the fraction absorbed into the hepatoportal circulation that escapes first-pass metabolism and from the administration of oral/parenteral corticosteroid (see Adverse Effects Focus, page 189).

The aims of asthma treatment are to control the disease and reduce the patient's symptoms whilst keeping the dose of corticosteroid to a minimum in order to minimise the risk of adverse effects. Only a minority of patients need long-term treatment with oral corticosteroids and in these patients drug therapy and asthma control should be reviewed regularly. The lowest possible dose that controls symptoms should be prescribed and it may be necessary to sacrifice complete control of symptoms in order to avoid toxicity.

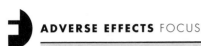

ADVERSE EFFECTS FOCUS

Side-effects of corticosteroid therapy

Inhaled treatment

- Adrenal suppression (high doses)
- Growth suppression (high doses)
- Bruising
- Reduced bone mineral density
- Cataract formation
- Local: dysphonia (hoarseness of voice), oropharyngeal candidiasis

Oral treatment

- Growth suppression
- Musculoskeletal: myopathy, osteoporosis, loss of muscle mass
- Metabolic disturbances: diabetes, hypokalaemia, adrenal suppression, hyperlipidaemia, cushingoid appearance, secondary amenorrhoea, erectile dysfunction, weight gain because of increased appetite
- Infective complications: increased susceptibility to infection, reactivation of infection, dissemination of live vaccine; a few patients on high doses of oral corticosteroids (>2 mg/kg/day) have developed severe or fatal disseminated varicella (chickenpox)
- Cardiovascular: hypertension, exacerbation of congestive cardiac failure, oedema
- Gastrointestinal tract: peptic ulceration, oesophagitis, pancreatitis, intestinal perforation
- Ocular: cataract formation, glaucoma
- Dermal thinning and bruising, hirsuitism
- Psychiatric disturbances

Local adverse effects

Although the risk of adverse effects is lower with the inhaled route compared with the oral route, some side-effects do occur. As mentioned above, much of the dose of an ICS does not actually reach the lungs but is deposited instead in the mouth, where its effects in suppressing the immune system can lead to dysphonia (hoarseness of the voice) and allow thrush (*Candida albicans*) to develop. The risk of thrush depends on the dose of steroid and frequency of administration and on the delivery system used; clinical thrush occurs in only about 5% of patients on low-dose therapy but as many as 35% on high doses.[15] It is more common in adults than children. Use of a spacer or holding-chamber device and mouth washing (rinse with water, gargle and spit out) after inhalation can help prevent oral candidiasis.

The most frequent complaint is dysphonia, which affects 5–50% of patients (depending on the dose of corticosteroids used).[16] Using a spacer device does not totally reduce dysphonia, and the patient may need to switch to a dry-powder device if not already prescribed. Dysphonia may result from myopathy of the laryngeal muscles and is reversible on discontinuation of treatment.

Some people experience a reflex cough and bronchospasm following inhalation (particularly with the HFA-based inhalers); this can be reduced by breathing in more slowly and/or using a spacer device. These symptoms are likely to be caused by surfactants in pressurised aerosols, as they disappear after switching to a dry-powder inhaler device.

Systemic adverse effects

The efficacy of ICSs in the control of asthma is now established but there are concerns about the systemic effects of ICSs, particularly in children and when high inhaled doses are needed. Systemic adverse effects from ICSs are uncommon but may occur depending on several factors, including the dose delivered to the patient, the site of delivery (gastrointestinal tract and lung), the delivery system used, the corticosteroid inhaled and individual differences in patients' responses to the corticosteroid.

The systemic effect of an ICS depends on the amount of drug absorbed into the systemic circulation. Approximately 90% of the dose inhaled from a metered-dose inhaler (MDI) is deposited in the oropharynx and can be swallowed and subsequently absorbed from the gastrointestinal tract, potentially causing adverse effects. The use of a large-volume spacer device in conjunction with an MDI markedly reduces this deposition and the risk of subsequent adverse effects. It is therefore recommended that any patient prescribed a daily dose of greater than 800 micrograms of an ICS (beclometasone or equivalent) should be advised to use a spacer device.[3] With dry-powder inhalers, systemic effects can be reduced by mouth washing and discarding the fluid. The risk of systemic adverse effects is reduced when the oral bioavailability of the drug is low, as with fluticasone, which has a high first-pass metabolism. Even so, adverse effects can still occur, as approximately 10% of an ICS enters the lungs and this fraction can still be absorbed into the systemic circulation from the lungs. Indeed, flutisasone has been shown to cause adrenal suppression. Although this is a well-established dose-related adverse effect of all ICSs, it is observed more frequently with fluticasone, possibly because higher-than-licensed doses are widely prescribed. All ICSs are associated with an increased risk of systemic adverse effects when used at higher-than-licensed doses.[17] Whilst ICSs have a more favourable side-effect profile than systemic steroids, they are not free from adverse effects. The dose of ICS used should be carefully monitored, and kept at the lowest dose necessary to maintain adequate control of the patient's asthma.

The risk of systemic adverse effects from oral corticosteroids is well documented. Adverse effects depend on the dosage and duration of treatment, so patients should be given treatment for the shortest length of time at the lowest dose that is clinically necessary. Short rescue courses of oral corticosteroids (40–50 mg prednisolone daily for 5 days or until recovery) are indicated for exacerbations of asthma.[3] In this situation, the benefits of corticosteroid treatment in controlling the asthma far outweigh the possible adverse effects.

Oral corticosteroids are usually given as a single morning dose, as this reduces the risk of adverse effects because it coincides with the peak diurnal concentrations of cortisol. Systemic corticosteroids administered in the evening are more likely to cause clinically significant adrenal suppression.[18]

Reported systemic adverse effects include fluid retention, weight gain because of increased appetite, osteoporosis, skin thinning, bruising, hypertension, cataract formation, diabetes, peptic ulceration, adrenal suppression and psychosis.

Growth suppression

One of the most important potential systemic effects of corticosteroids is on children's growth, particularly as ICSs are likely to be used for several years. However, it is not clear whether long-term use of an ICS does affect growth significantly. It is likely that the higher the dose the more likely it is to affect growth but then asthma itself can affect growth and delay puberty. Longitudinal studies have demonstrated that ICSs have no significant effect on statural growth in doses of up to 800 micrograms daily (beclometasone or equivalent) and up to 5 years of treatment.[19,20] Growth suppression can certainly occur if very high doses of corticosteroids (i.e. >1000 micrograms fluticasone daily) are inhaled. It is therefore important to monitor growth in children taking an ICS long term by regularly plotting the child's height and weight on centile charts. Those prescribed a high maintenance dose should be reviewed regularly by a paediatrician.

Musculoskeletal effects

Corticosteroids can affect bone density, which might predispose to osteoporosis and fractures. The effects of oral corticosteroids on osteoporosis and increased risk of vertebral and rib fractures are well known. Oral corticosteroids significantly increase the risk of spine and hip fracture, even at doses less than 7.5 mg prednisolone per day. The rate of bone mineral density (BMD) loss is greatest in the first few months of corticosteroid use.[21]

Patients with asthma taking oral steroids for more than 3 months should be offered osteoporosis prophylaxis if they are over 65 years of age or have had a previous fragility fracture (i.e. occurring after the age of 40 years or with minimal trauma).[21]

In other individuals, it is recommended that the BMD is measured using dual energy X-ray absorptiometry to access the fracture risk. Osteoporosis prophylaxis should be considered if the T score is −1.5 or lower. Patients taking intermittent courses of oral corticosteroids over longer periods of time should have their BMD monitored. There is some evidence that bone loss is related to cumulative doses of corticosteroids.

It is not known whether long-term use of lower doses of ICSs has osteoporotic effects, but there is evidence that doses over 800 micrograms daily (beclometasone or equivalent) may do so. Although there is evidence that BMD may be reduced in patients taking ICSs, interpretation is confounded by the fact that many of these patients also receive intermittent courses of oral corticosteroids. Elderly women are most likely to suffer these effects as they are at risk of osteoporosis and fracture without the complication of taking steroids. However, the risks of uncontrolled asthma outweigh the possible disadvantages of the ICSs in this regard, and short-term oral steroid treatment should not present a problem. General measures to counteract osteoporosis (such as regular exercise, smoking cessation, adequate dietary calcium) are prudent in people who require high doses of ICSs for prolonged periods of time.[21]

Muscle wasting and a degree of myopathy occurs in many patients on long-term corticosteroids. This is a particular problem in patients ventilated for acute severe asthma and treated with intravenous hydrocortisone.

Metabolic effects

Electrolyte imbalance, particularly hypokalaemia, can be a problem, as patients may also be receiving high-dose inhaled beta-2 agonists and methylxanthines (e.g. theophylline), which also lower plasma potassium levels. Plasma potassium concentrations should therefore be monitored carefully.

Diabetes may be unmasked or exacerbated in patients receiving high doses of oral corticosteroids. The diabetes will usually resolve when the steroids are stopped. Plasma glucose levels should be monitored in patients at risk of developing diabetes and also in those patients with existing diabetes, as the addition of a corticosteroid may increase blood sugar levels.

The cushingoid appearance and weight gain is a side-effect that causes patients considerable anxiety. Steroids cause weight gain mainly by an increase in appetite, with a minor contribution from fluid retention. There is also redistribution of body mass from the peripheries to the centre. Patients should receive dietary advice at the start of oral corticosteroid treatment, as weight gain is easier to prevent than to reverse.

Corticosteroids may cause suppression of the hypothalamic–pituitary–adrenal (HPA) axis by reducing production of corticotrophin (ACTH), which reduces cortisol secretion by the adrenal gland. The degree of suppression depends on the dose, duration, frequency and timing of corticosteroid administration. Studies have shown that doses of ICSs less than 1500 micrograms in adults and less than 400 micrograms in children (beclometasone or equivalent) have no significant suppressive effects on the HPA axis. The adrenal atrophy that may develop can persist for years after stopping the steroid.

Abrupt withdrawal after a prolonged period may lead to acute adrenal insufficiency, hypotension or death. Withdrawal may also be associated with fever, myalgia, arthralgia, rhinitis, conjunctivitis, painful itchy skin nodules and weight loss. After prolonged oral therapy, the dose of oral corticosteroid must therefore be reduced slowly.[22]

To compensate for any reduction in adrenocortisol response secondary to prolonged steroid treatment, any significant intercurrent illness, trauma or surgical procedure requires a temporary increase in corticosteroid dose. Patients taking long-term steroids should carry a steroid treatment card, which provides guidance on minimising risk and gives details on drug, dosage and duration of treatment.

Infection

Oral corticosteroids may mask the signs and symptoms of an infection such that serious infections (e.g. tuberculosis and septicaemia) may reach an advanced stage before being recognised. Prolonged courses of corticosteroids may also increase susceptibility to infections and the severity of infections.

A small number of cases have been reported of patients on high doses of oral corticosteroids (>2 mg/kg/day) developing severe or fatal disseminated varicella (chickenpox). Patients who have not had chickenpox and who are taking oral or parenteral corticosteroids for purposes other than replacement should be regarded as being at high risk and should be treated appropriately.

Cardiovascular effects

Development of mild-to-moderate hypertension or exacerbation of existing hypertension are extremely common adverse effects relating to the long-term use of oral corticosteroids. Patients should be monitored and treated accordingly.

Fluid retention and peripheral oedema are particular problems in elderly patients who may have coexisting heart disease. Low doses of potassium-sparing diuretics are usually sufficient to control this.

Gastrointestinal tract effects

Many patients complain of gastric irritation when taking oral prednisolone. This can be reduced by encouraging patients to take tablets with food. The association of oral corticosteroids steroids with peptic ulceration and gastrointestinal haemorrhage is controversial, with conflicting results from studies. The benefit of prescribing anti-ulcer drugs in patients taking oral steroids is therefore debatable unless the patient has other risk factors for gastrointestinal complications.

Ocular effects

There is no evidence that ICSs increase the risk of cataract formation at normal doses but long-term, high-dose treatment may increase the risk of cataract formation and also of glaucoma. Patients with an existing predisposition to glaucoma should be monitored.

Other effects

Other systemic side-effects, such as dermal thinning, easy skin bruising and hirsuitism, have been reported in elderly patients receiving high doses of an ICS, frequent courses of oral steroids or long-term maintenance doses. The risk depends on the dosage, route of administration and duration of treatment, as well as on the age of the patient.

There have been rare reports of psychiatric disturbances secondary to high-dose oral steroids. These include emotional lability, euphoria, depression, aggressiveness and insomnia.

Drug interactions

Antacids

The absorption of oral prednisolone can be reduced by large doses of aluminium or magnesium hydroxide antacids.[23]

Liver enzyme inducers

The clearance of prednisolone from the body is increased by drugs that induce the liver cytochrome P450 enzymes, for example phenobarbital, carbamazepine, phenytoin and rifampicin, necessitating an increase in the dose of oral steroids.[23]

Diuretics

Both corticosteroids and diuretics cause potassium loss and severe depletion may occur if they are used together. The use of potassium-sparing diuretics may help to avoid this complication.[23]

Live vaccines

Patients who are immunised with live vaccines while receiving immunosuppressive doses of corticosteroids may develop generalised, possibly life-threatening, infections. The *British National Formulary* recommends that live vaccination should be postponed for at least 3 months after stopping high-dose corticosteroids.[22]

Preparations

The preparations, dosages and indications of corticosteroids used in the treatment of asthma are summarised in Table 12.2.

Table 12.2 Routes of administration, recommended dosages, indications and preparations of corticosteroids used in the treatment of asthma

Corticosteroid	Route of administration	Recommended dosage[3,19]	Indication and Comments	UK proprietary name(s) (Manufacturer)
Beclometasone dipropionate	Aerosol inhalation, breath-actuated inhalation, dry-powder for inhalation	*Adults:* 200 mcg twice daily (adjust dose according to symptoms) or 100 mcg three or four times daily (twice-daily dosing recommended by BTS/SIGN) *Children:* 50–100 mcg 2–4 times daily QVAR 50–200 mcg twice daily, increased to maximum of 400 mcg twice daily if necessary	Prophylaxis of asthma	*Aerosol* Non-proprietary (APS, Generics) Beclazone (IVAX) Becotide (A&H) QVAR (IVAX) AeroBec Forte (3M) Becloforte (A&H) ***Breath-actuated inhalation*** Beclazone Easi-Breathe (IVAX) AeroBec Autohaler (3M) QVAR autohaler (IVAX) ***Dry powder for inhalation*** Pulvinal (Trinity) Beclometasone Cyclocaps (APS) Asmabec Clickhaler (Celltech) Becodisks (A&H)
Budesonide	Aerosol inhalation	*Adults:* 200 mcg twice daily, may be reduced in well-controlled asthma to not less than 200 mcg daily; may be increased to 1.6 mg daily in severe asthma *Children:* 50–400 mcg twice daily; may be increased to 800 mcg daily in severe asthma	Prophylaxis of asthma	Pulmicort (AstraZeneca) Pulmicort LS (AstraZeneca)

Corticosteroid	Route of administration	Recommended dosage[3,19]	Indication and Comments	UK proprietary name(s) (Manufacturer)
	Dry powder for inhalation	*Adult:* when starting treatment, during periods of severe asthma and while reducing or discontinuing oral corticosteroid, 200 mcg to 1.6 mg daily in two divided doses; in less severe cases 200–400 mcg once daily (evening); patients whose symptoms are already controlled on inhaled beclometasone or budesonide twice daily may be transferred to once-daily dosing at the same equivalent total daily dose *Child under 12 years:* 200–800 mcg daily in two divided doses		Pulmicort Turbohaler (AstraZeneca) Novolizer (Viatris)
	Nebulised solution for inhalation	*Adults:* When starting treatment, during periods of severe asthma and while reducing or discontinuing oral corticosteroid, 1–2 mg twice daily (may be increased further in severe asthma) *Children aged 3 months – 12 years:* 0.5–1 mg twice daily Maintenance usually half the above doses	Patients unable to use an inhaler combined with a spacer with or without a facemask	Pulmicort Respules (AstraZeneca)

Symbicort (Budesonide with formoterol)	Dry-powder inhalation	100/6
		  One or two puffs twice daily, increased if necessary up to a maximum of 4 inhalations twice daily
		Adolescents aged 12–17 years: one or two puffs twice daily
		Children aged over 6 years: two puffs twice daily
		Not recommended for children under 6 years
		200/6
		  One or two puffs twice daily, increased if necessary to a maximum of four puffs twice daily, reduced to one puff once daily if control is maintained
		Adolescents aged 12–17 years: one or two puffs twice daily reduced to one puff once daily if control is maintained
		Not recommended for children under 12 years
		400/12
		  One or two puffs twice daily, reduced to one puff once daily if control is maintained
		Adolescents aged 12–17 years: one puff twice daily reduced to one puff once daily if control is maintained
		Not recommended for children under 12 years
			Prophylaxis of asthma	Symbicort Turbohaler (AstraZeneca)

Continued

Table 12.2 Continued

Corticosteroid	Route of administration	Recommended dosage[3,19]	Indication and Comments	UK proprietary name(s) (Manufacturer)
Fluticasone propionate	Aerosol inhalation, dry powder for inhalation	**Adults and children over 16 years:** 100–250 mcg twice daily, increased according to severity of asthma to 1 mg twice daily (note that the maximum licensed dose is not recommended by the BTS/SIGN asthma guidelines) **Children aged 4–16 years:** 50–100 mcg twice daily, adjusted as necessary; maximum 200 mcg twice daily	Prophylaxis of asthma	*Aerosol* Flixotide Evohaler (A&H) *Dry powder inhalers* Flixotide Accuhaler (A&H) Flixotide Diskhaler (A&H)
	Nebulised solution for inhalation	**Adults and children over 16 years:** 0.5–2 mg twice daily **Children 4–16 years:** 1 mg twice daily	Patients unable to use an inhaler combined with a spacer with or without a facemask	Flixotide Nebules (A&H)
Seretide (fluticasone with salmeterol)	Aerosol inhalation	**Adults and children over 4 years** *Seretide 50:* two puffs twice daily, reduced to two puffs once daily if control is maintained **Adults and children over 12 years** *Seretide 125:* two puffs twice daily *Seretide 250:* two puffs twice daily	Regular long-term treatment of moderate reversible airways obstruction	Seretide Evohaler (A&H)
	Dry powder inhalation	**Adults and children over 4 years** *Accuhaler 100:* one blister twice daily, reduced to one blister once daily if control is maintained **Adults and children over 12 years** *Accuhaler 250:* one blister twice daily *Accuhaler 500:* one blister twice daily	Regular long-term treatment of moderate reversible airways obstruction	Seretide Accuhaler (A&H)
Mometasone furoate	Dry powder for inhalation	**Adults and children over 12 years** 200–400 mcg as a single dose in the evening or in two divided doses; increased to 400 mcg twice daily if necessary Not recommended for children under 12 years	Prophylaxis of asthma	Asmanex Twisthaler (Schering-Plough)
Ciclesonide	Aerosol inhalation	**Adults and children over 12 years** 160 mcg once daily (evening); can be reduced to 80 mcg once daily if asthma is stable Not recommended for children under 12 years	Prophylaxis of asthma	Alvesco (Altana)

A&H, Allen & Hanbury; BTS/SIGN, British Thoracic Society/Scottish Intercollegiate Guidelines Network asthma management guideline;[3] mcg, micrograms.

References

1. O'Byrne PM, Barnes PJ, Rodriguez-Roisin R, *et al.* Low dose inhaled budesonide and formoterol in mild persistent asthma: the OPTIMA randomized trial. *Am J Respir Crit Care Med* 2001; 164: 1392–1397.
2. Pauwels RA, Pedersen S, Busse WW, *et al.* Early intervention with budesonide in mild persistent asthma: a randomised, double-blind trial. *Lancet* 2003; 361(9363): 1071–1076.
3. British Thoracic Society/Scottish Intercollegiate Guidelines Network. British Guideline on the Management of Asthma. *Thorax* 2003; 58 (Suppl I): S1–S94.
4. Barnes PJ. Anti-inflammatory actions of glucocorticoids: molecular mechanisms. *Clin Sci* 1998; 94: 557–572.
5. Barnes PJ, Adcock IM. Transcription factors and asthma. *Eur Respir J* 1998; 12: 221–234.
6. Mak JCW, Nishikawa M, Shirasaki H, *et al.* Protective effects of a glucocorticoid on down-regulation of pulmonary beta-2–adrenergic receptors in vivo. *J Clin Invest* 1995; 96: 99–106.
7. Barnes PJ, Pedersen S, Busse WW. Efficacy and safety of inhaled corticosteroids: an update. *Am J Respir Crit Care Med* 1998; 157: S1–S53.
8. Derendorf H. Relevant pharmacokinetic parameters for determining efficacy and safety in inhaled corticosteroids. *Eur Respir Rev* 2004; 13: 62–65.
9. Pharmacological management of asthma. Evidence table 4.7: high dose step down. Edinburgh: SIGN; 2002. Available from: http: //www.sign.ac.uk/ guidelines/published/support/guideline63/index.html.
10. Greening AP, Ind PW, Northfield M, *et al.* Additional salmeterol versus higher dose corticosteroid in asthma patients with symptoms on existing inhaled corticosteroid. *Lancet* 1994; 344: 219–224.
11. Woolcock A, Lundback B, Ringdal N, *et al.* Comparison of addition of salmeterol in inhaled corticosteroids with doubling the dose of inhaled corticosteroids. *Am J Respir Crit Care Med* 1996; 153: 1481–1488.
12. Pauwels RA, Lofdahl C-G, Postma DS, *et al.* Effect of inhaled formoterol and budesonide on exacerbations of asthma. *N Engl J Med* 1997; 337: 1412–1418.
13. Jones AH, Langdon CG, Lee PS, *et al.* Pulmicort Turbohaler once daily as initial prophylactic therapy for asthma. *Resp Med* 1994; 88: 293–299.
14. Engel T, Heninig JH. Glucocorticoid therapy in acute severe asthma – a critical review. *Eur Respir J* 1991; 4: 881–889.
15. Toogood JA, Jennings B, Greenway RW, *et al.* Candidiasis and dysphonia complicating beclometasone treatment of asthma. *J Allergy Clin Immunol* 1980; 65: 145–153.
16. Williamson IJ, Matusiewicz SP, Brwon PH, *et al.* Frequency of voice problems and cough in patients using pressurised aerosol inhaled corticosteroid preparations. *Eur Resp J* 1995; 8: 590–592.
17. Committee on Safety of Medicines (CSM)/Medicines Control Agency (MCA). Inhaled corticosteroids and adrenal suppression in children. *Curr Prob Pharmacovigilance* 2002; 28: 7.
18. Committee on Safety of Medicines (CSM)/Medicines Control Agency (MCA). Focus on corticosteroids. *Curr Prob Pharmacovigilance* 1998; 24: 1–6.

19. Volovitz B, Malik H, Kauschansky A, *et al.* Growth and pituitary-adrenal function in children with severe asthma traeted with inhaled budesonide. *N Engl J Med* 1993; 329: 1703–1708.
20. Allen DB, Mullen M, Mullen B. A meta-analysis of the effects of oral and inhaled corticosteroids on growth. *J Allergy Clin Immunol* 1994; 93: 967–976.
21. Royal College of Physicians of London. *Glucocorticoid-induced Osteoporosis*. London: Royal College of Physicians, 2003. www.rcplondon.ac.uk/pubs/books/glucocorticoid/index.asp
22. British Medical Association/Royal Pharmaceutical Society of Great Britain. *British National Formulary* 51. London: BMJ Publishing Group/RPS Publishing, March 2006.
23. Baxter K (ed.). Stockley's *Drug Interactions*, 7th edn. London: Pharmaceutical Press, 2006.

13

Methylxanthines

Indications

In 1886, Henry Hyde Salter described the efficacious use of strong coffee taken on an empty stomach as a treatment of asthma.[1] Methylxanthines (theophylline and aminophylline; Figure 13.1), which are related to caffeine, have been used in the treatment of asthma since the 1930s. They are mild bronchodilators that are taken orally. Although theophylline and aminophylline are still used to treat asthma, they are less potent and much more toxic than inhaled beta-2 agonists and the need for serum monitoring involves taking frequent blood samples, which is inconvenient and is particularly unsuitable for children.

As it has a long duration of action, sustained-release theophylline is mostly used to treat nocturnal asthma symptoms that occur despite treatment with corticosteroids, although it is less effective than the long-acting beta-2 agonists.[2] Also, if taken before sleep, theophylline may cause insomnia. Nowadays, therefore, theophylline is reserved for use in severe asthma when inhaled corticosteroids and beta-2 agonists (both long and short acting) have failed to control symptoms.[3]

Mechanism of action

Even though theophylline has been in clinical use for many years, its mechanism of action is still uncertain and several modes of action have been proposed:

- inhibition of phosphodiesterase
- adenosine receptor antagonist
- stimulation of catecholamine release
- inhibition of the degranulation and release of mediators, including platelet-activating factor and leukotriene C4, from eosinophils and granulocytes *in vitro*
- inhibition of intracellular calcium release.

Xanthine

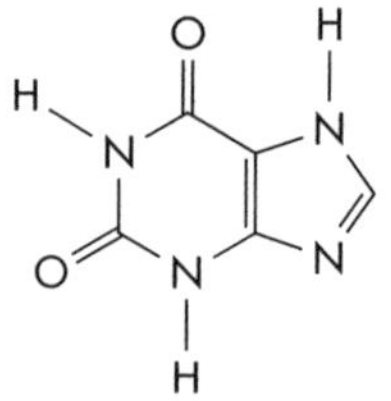

Caffeine

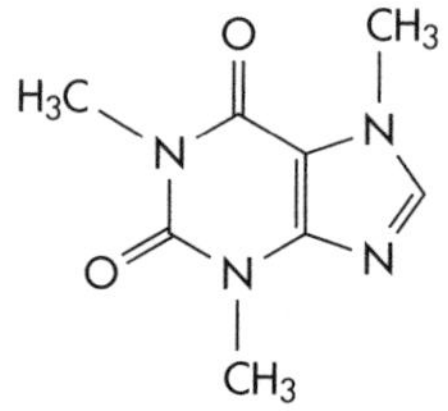

Theophylline

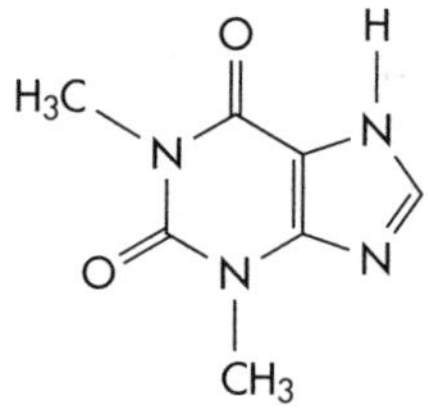

Aminophylline

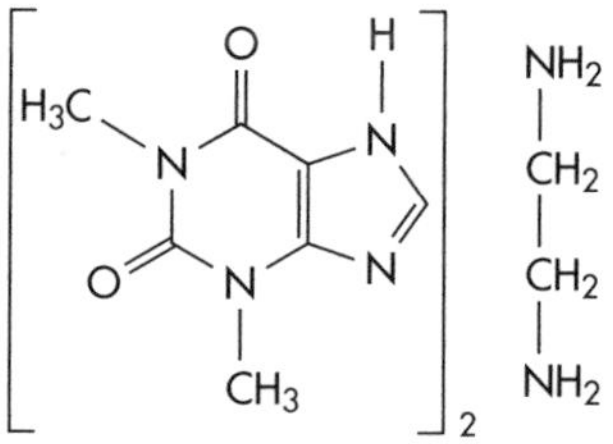

Figure 13.1 Chemical structures of xanthine and derivatives. The natural metabolite is xanthine, which is a precursor of uric acid. Theophylline and caffeine are methylated xanthine derivatives. Aminophylline (a mixture of theophylline with ethylenediamine) is converted to theophylline by the liver.

Whilst theophylline has traditionally been classed as a bronchodilator, it is becoming increasingly apparent that this drug has a range of other pharmacological effects that occur independently of the bronchodilator actions, including anti-inflammatory and immunomodulatory actions and stimulation of respiratory drive.

Methylxanthines promote bronchial smooth muscle relaxation, increase mucociliary transport and diaphragmatic contractility and stimulate central respiratory drive. They are thought to cause bronchodilation either by interfering with the chemical mechanism by which smooth muscle contracts, by inhibiting the action of phosphodiesterase, thus raising the intracellular levels of cyclic adenosine monophosphate (cAMP) (see Figure 13.2),[4] and/or they prevent adenosine (a natural bronchoconstrictor) from binding to the smooth muscle cells by blocking adenosine receptors. Although adenosine acts as a bronchoconstrictor in patients with asthma, it is not clear whether adenosine has a pathophysiological role in asthma. Blocking of adenosine receptors may account for some of the side-effects of theophylline, such as central nervous system stimulation, cardiac arrhythmias and diuresis. Interestingly, in overdose, symptoms of both beta-1 and beta-2 adrenoceptor agonist activity are seen. This may be secondary to an increase in adrenaline (epinephrine) from the adrenal medulla. However, this increase in plasma adrenaline concentration is small and is insufficient to account for any significant bronchodilator effect.[5] These molecular mechanisms of action produce a number of clinical responses (see Monitoring Focus, page 204).

Pharmacokinetics

Serum theophylline levels

Theophylline has a narrow therapeutic index and serum theophylline concentrations must be monitored carefully in order to avoid potentially

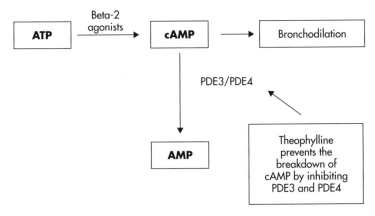

Figure 13.2 Inhibition of the phosphodiesterases (PDEs) by theophylline. ATP, adenosine, triphosphate; cAMP, cyclic adenosine monophosphate AMP, a denosine monophosphate.

MONITORING FOCUS

Clinical effects of theophylline
• Bronchodilation • Lung deflation and reduction in residual volume • Improvement in diaphragmatic and respiratory muscles • Increased mucociliary clearance[6] • Anti-inflammatory effects

serious adverse effects. Most textbooks state that serum theophylline concentrations need to be maintained in the range 10–20 mg/litre. However, the concentration required for effective therapy is 5–15 mg/litre and the optimal range is quoted as 10–12 mg/litre.[7] Adverse effects can occur within this range but above 10–20 mg/litre, progressively more serious side-effects are likely (see Monitoring Focus, below). The non-bronchodilatory effects of theophylline often occur at plasma levels below 10 mg/litre, suggesting that lower levels of theophylline than have previously been used to obtain bronchodilation may be of benefit in the treatment of lung diseases, thus reducing the side-effect profile and improving the safety margin of the drug.[8] The therapeutic window has thus been reduced in many countries to 5–15 mg/litre.

Serum concentrations should be monitored when starting theophylline therapy, at regular intervals afterwards and if the patient develops adverse events, does not respond to treatment or if conditions known to affect serum levels occur. Serum theophylline levels are best

MONITORING FOCUS

Serum theophylline concentrations	
Theophylline serum concentration (mg/litre)	**Clinical effect**
>30	Seizures
>25	Cardiac arrhythmias
>20	Nausea and vomiting
10–20	Therapeutic range
(5–15 in some countries)	
10–12	Optimal range
<5	No bronchodilator effects seen

measured at the time of peak absorption of the drug, this being 5–9 hours after the morning dose of sustained-release theophylline.

The dosage of theophylline can be adjusted using the theophylline dosage adjustment guide (see Management Focus, below).

Factors affecting theophylline blood levels

Theophylline is readily absorbed from the gastrointestinal tract, but many factors affect the metabolism of theophylline by the liver and hence can alter the concentration of theophylline in the blood. Theophylline is mainly metabolised in the liver by the cytochrome P450 enzymes, in particular CYP1A2. Some cytochrome P450 enzymes are susceptible to induction and inhibition by various environmental factors and drugs (see Risk Factors Focus, page 206). CYP1A2 is highly inducible by a number of chemicals, including many found in cigarette smoke, and this may contribute to the wide variability in the metabolism of theophylline. Patients with asthma who smoke may have high levels of CYP1A2 and

MANAGEMENT FOCUS

Theophylline dosage adjustment guide	
Serum concentration (mg/litre)	**Action**
Too high	
20–25	Decrease dose by 10%
25–30	Skip next dose and decrease subsequent doses by 25%; check plasma concentration
>30	Skip next two doses and decrease subsequent doses by 50%; check plasma concentration
Therapeutic	
10–20	• Maintain dosage if tolerated • Check plasma concentration every 6–12 months
Too low	
7.5–10	Increase dose by 25%
5–7.5	Increase dose by 25%; check concentration

Notes
- Increase dosage in patients whose condition is not well controlled.
- Ensure peak plasma concentration is measured appropriately.

may therefore require higher doses than non-smokers. Dose adjustment would be required in patients who stop smoking. In general, only a 20% or greater inhibition or a 50% or greater induction of theophylline metabolism is likely to result in a clinically significant interaction.

Theophylline is water soluble and does not distribute into fatty tissues; hence ideal body weight should be used in calculating theophylline dosages (see Management Focus, page 207). Theophylline is largely eliminated by the kidneys.

Dosage

Oral theophylline

In attempts to reduce the incidence of adverse effects from theophylline, the drug has been formulated in a variety of sustained-release

RISK FACTORS FOCUS

Factors that affect theophylline metabolism	
Factors that increase metabolism (i.e. decrease plasma concentration); dose increase therefore required	Smoking tobacco, marijuana Chronic alcoholism Childhood Barbecued meat High-protein, low-carbohydrate diet Enzyme induction: rifampicin, phenobarbital, anticonvulsants
Factors that decrease metabolism (i.e. increase plasma concentration) dose reduction therefore required	Heart failure, including cor pulmonale Cirrhosis/liver disease Bacterial infections (e.g. pneumonia) Viral hepatitis Old age Respiratory acidosis Obesity Vaccination High-carbohydrate diet Enzyme inhibition: cimetidine (not ranitidine), ciprofloxacin, erythromycin, allopurinol, fluvoxamine, propranolol, oral contraceptives, zafirlukast (see Adverse Effects Focus on page 211 for more details)

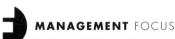

Ideal body weight (IBW)

IBW (in kg) is the weight expected for a non-obese person of a given height, which can be calculated using the formulas below.

Adults (aged 18 years and older)[9]	**Men:** 50 + (2.3 × height in inches over 5 feet) **Women:** 45.5 + (2.3 × height in inches over 5 feet)
Children (aged 1–<18 years)[10]	
Children under 5 feet tall	IBW = (height^2 × 1.65) / 1000 where IBW is in kg and height is in cm
Children 5 feet or taller	**Boys:** 39 + (2.27 × height in inches over 5 feet) **Girls:** 42.2 + (2.27 × height in inches over 5 feet) where IBW is in kg

preparations (see Table 13.1). These preparations maintain relatively constant serum concentrations and should be taken twice daily. The degree of fluctuation in serum theophylline concentrations over the dosing interval in any particular patient depends on the release characteristics of the product and the elimination characteristics in that patient. Thus, given the same product over the same dosing interval, patients in whom clearance of theophylline is rapid (e.g. smokers) will experience greater fluctuations than patients in whom clearance is slow.

For long-term use, the dose of oral theophylline should be increased slowly in increments (see Management Focus, page 208).

Intravenous aminophylline

Aminophylline is a mixture of theophylline with ethylenediamine, which is 20 times more soluble than theophylline alone, and is administered intravenously to patients with acute severe asthma. This should always be done with care, especially in patients who have been taking oral theophylline or aminophylline, since the concentration of drug may already be high at admission. Aminophylline is metabolised to theophylline in the liver.

MANAGEMENT FOCUS 13.3

Long-term oral dosing with theophylline
All recommendations are based on the average theophylline clearance for a given population.

Initial starting dose	200 mg every 12 hours for 1 week
Week 2	Increase dose to 300 mg every 12 hours for 1 week
Week 3	Increase dose to 400 mg every 12 hours

Notes

- Every week the dose can be adjusted by 100–150 mg steps according to serum blood concentrations. Depending on the formulation and manufacturer's recommendations, the maximum dose may eventually be 500 mg every 12 hours.
- A larger evening dose or morning dose can be given to provide an increase in drug concentration when the patient's symptoms are worse. However, increasing the evening dose may cause sleep disturbances.

For acute severe asthma, an intravenous loading dose is required to optimise serum levels. This should only be administered if the patient has not received any oral theophylline or aminophylline in the previous 24 hours. A suitable dose is 5 mg/kg, based on the patient's ideal body weight if they are obese (see Management Focus, page 207). Injections should be given slowly, because of the cardiotoxicity of the drug. The asthma management guideline published by the British Thoracic Society (BTS) and Scottish Intercollegiate Guidelines Network[3] recommends electrocardiogram monitoring in patients naive to theophylline. After the initial loading dose, an intravenous infusion should be started to maintain an adequate serum concentration. If the patient has taken any amount of oral theophylline then the serum theophylline concentration should be measured before the infusion is initiated, to guide the dose. However, if symptoms are severe and there is no clinical evidence of toxicity, the maintenance infusion should be started and the plasma theophylline concentration checked 4–6 hours later. The recommended maintenance dose is 500 micrograms/kg/hour.[11]

Contraindications and special precautions for use

Contraindications to methylxanthines include porphyria, hypersensitivity to any of the product constituents and concomitant administration with ephedrine in children.

Smoking and alcohol consumption can increase the clearance of theophylline and a higher dose may be necessary. Careful monitoring is recommended for patients with congestive heart failure, chronic alcoholism, hepatic dysfunction, or viral infections, as they may have a lower clearance of theophylline, which could lead to higher-than-normal plasma levels. Caution should be exercised in patients with peptic ulcer, cardiac arrhythmia other cardiovascular diseases, hyperthyroidism or hypertension. The use of alternative treatments is advised in patients with a history of seizures, as these may be exacerbated by theophylline.

Adverse effects

Adverse effects of methylxanthines are usually related to plasma concentrations and tend to occur when plasma levels exceed 20 mg/litre. Some patients may experience adverse effects when the drug is initiated or the dose is increased; this can be reduced by gradually increasing the dose until the therapeutic concentrations are achieved.

Gastrointestinal symptoms (nausea and vomiting) are the most common side-effects, but severe symptoms (seizures and even death) can occur without warning, and ingestion of as little as 4.5 g can be fatal. Gastrointestinal symptoms can be transient and may diminish after 2–3 days continued treatment but they may be intolerable to some patients, even well within the usual therapeutic drug range.

Different preparations of theophylline are absorbed to different extents, so the manufacturer's instructions should be used as a guide to establishing the correct therapeutic dose. It is important that a patient's brand of tablet is not changed without careful monitoring. The Adverse Effects Focus on page 210 gives the potential adverse effects of theophylline and derivatives.

Drug interactions

Theophylline and aminophylline are subject to many drug and disease interactions (see the Risk Factors Focus on page 211). The hepatic cytochrome P450 enzymes that metabolise theophylline, particularly CYP1A2, are susceptible to induction and inhibition; a 20% or greater

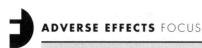

ADVERSE EFFECTS FOCUS

Adverse effects of theophylline and its derivatives
• Nausea and vomiting, loss of appetite, gastric upset, abdominal discomfort, heartburn, gastro-oesophageal reflux, diarrhoea, haematemesis
• Headache, anxiety, restlessness, insomnia, tremor
• Epileptic seizures (including grand mal episodes)
• Diuresis
• Cardiac: arrhythmias, palpitations, atrial and ventricular arrhythmias, supraventricular tachycardia, ventricular tachycardia
• Hypotension

inhibition or 50% or greater induction of metabolism is likely to result in clinically significant interactions. There is a significant interpatient susceptibility to developing an interaction. It is essential that health professionals are aware of the potential drug interactions so that appropriate precautions and actions can be taken.[11,12]

The Medicines and Healthcare products Regulatory Agency (MHRA) has advised that caution is required in patients with severe asthma, as the hypokalaemic effect of beta-2 agonists may be potentiated by aminophylline. Plasma potassium levels should be monitored in patients with severe asthma.

Preparations

Many different sustained-release formulations of theophylline and aminophylline are available (see Table 13.1) and these differ in pharmacokinetic profile. Caution should be taken when switching a patient from one sustained-release preparation to another and should be avoided if possible. The Council of the Royal Pharmaceutical Society of Great Britain advises pharmacists that if a general practitioner prescribes a sustained-release theophylline preparation without specifying a brand name, the pharmacist should agree the brand to be dispensed with the prescriber. Similarly, when patients are discharged from hospital, it is essential that they are maintained on the brand on which they were stabilised as in-patients.[11]

Aminophylline is the parenteral form of theophylline. It is a mixture of theophylline with ethylenediamine, which is 20 times more soluble than theophylline alone, and is used for severe attacks of asthma. It must be given by slow intravenous injection.

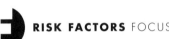

Significant drug interactions with theophylline[11,12]

Cimetidine	Cimetidine inhibits the metabolism of theophylline, decreasing clearance by 20–40%; this interaction has been reported to cause severe theophylline toxicity, including vomiting, seizures and death
Macrolide antibiotics	Erythromycin inhibits the metabolism of theophylline, decreasing clearance by 10–40%; the effect is time-dependent and is seen with erythromycin treatment for longer than 5 days
	The dose of theophylline should be reduced by 25% on beginning treatment with erythromycin
Rifampicin	Rifampicin induces theophylline metabolism, increasing the clearance by up to 80%
	The dose of theophylline should be increased by about 25% on starting rifampicin and reduced by half when rifampicin is stopped
	Careful monitoring of plasma theophylline concentrations is essential
Anticonvulsants	Phenytoin and carbamazepine increase theophylline clearance by up to 70%
	Patients taking either of these two drugs will require higher doses of theophylline to have the desired effect
	Plasma theophylline concentrations should be monitored carefully
	Phenobarbital can also increase theophylline clearance by inducing cytochrome P450 enzymes.
Allopurinol	At a dose of 300 mg/day for 7 days, allopurinol does not alter theophylline clearance; higher doses (600 mg daily for 14 days) decrease clearance by 20%
Antacids	Concomitant administration of antacids may affect the bioavailability or absorption characteristics of sustained-released preparations
Calcium channel blockers	Verapamil and diltiazem decrease theophylline clearance by 18% and 12%, respectively
Quinolone antibiotics	A number of quinolone antibiotics inhibit the metabolism of theophylline
	Ciprofloxacin can reduce the clearance of theophylline by 20–30%

Table 13.1 Methylxanthine preparations

UK brand (manufacturer)	Dosage
Oral theophylline: indicated for relief of acute asthma symptoms and for moderate-to severe-chronic asthma (Step 4 and above of the British Thoracic Society/Scottish Intercollegiate Guidelines Network asthma management guideline)	
Slo-Phyllin (Merck)	**Adults** 250–500 mg every 12 hours **Children** 2–6 years: 60–120 mg every 12 hours 7–12 years: 125–250 mg every 12 hours
Uniphyllin Continus (Napp)	**Adults** 200 mg every 12 hours, increased according to response to 400 mg every 12 hours **Children** 9 mg/kg twice daily; some children with chronic asthma may require 10–16 mg/kg every 12 hours
Nuelin SA (3M)	**SA tablets** **Adults:** 175–350 mg every 12 hours **Children over 6 years:** 175 mg every 12 hours **SA 250 tablets** **Adults:** 250–500 mg every 12 hours **Children over 6 years:** 125–250 mg every 12 hours
Oral aminophylline: indicated for reversible airways obstruction	
Aminophylline (non-proprietary) Phyllocontin Continus (225 mg) (Napp)	100–300 mg three or four times daily, after food One tablet twice daily initially, increased after 1 week to two tablets twice daily

UK brand (manufacturer)	Dosage
Amnivent 225 SR (Ashbourne) Norphylline SR (IVAX) Phyllocontin Forte tablets (350 mg) (Napp) (higher strength tablets suitable for smokers and other patients in whom theophylline half-life is decreased)	One tablet twice daily initially, increased after 1 week to two tablets twice daily – adjust according to theophylline blood concentration
Phyllocontin Paediatric tablets (100 mg) (Napp)	*Children over 3 years*: 6 mg/kg twice daily initially, increased after 1 week to 12 mg/kg twice daily; some children with chronic asthma may require 13–20 mg/kg every 12 hours

Intravenous aminophylline: indicated for acute severe asthma

Aminophylline (non-proprietary)	**For deteriorating acute severe asthma NOT previously treated with theophylline or aminophylline:** 250–500 mg (5 mg/kg) by slow intravenous injection over at least 20 minutes, then as for acute severe asthma *Children:* 5 mg/kg, then as for acute severe asthma **Acute severe asthma** 500 micrograms/kg/hour by intravenous infusion, adjusted according to plasma theophylline concentrations *Children aged 10–16 years*: 800 micrograms/kg/hour, adjusted according to plasma theophylline concentration *Children aged 6 months–9 year*: 1 mg/kg/hour, adjusted according to plasma theophylline concentrations Note: patients taking oral methylxanthines should not receive intravenous aminophylline unless plasma theophylline concentration is known, to guide dosage

Theophylline is included in some cough and decongestant preparations that are available as pharmacy medicines. Examples are Franol Plus and Do-Do Chesteze, both containing theophylline and ephedrine. These products must be avoided by patients who are taking theophylline or aminophylline.

References

1. Persson CG. On the medical history of xanthines and other remedies for asthma: a tribute to HH Salter. *Thorax* 1985; 40: 1183–1187.
2. Wiegand L, Mende CN, Zaidel G, *et al.* Salmeterol versus theophylline: Sleep and efficacy outcomes in patients with nocturnal asthma. *Chest* 1999; 115: 1525–1532.
3. British Thoracic Society/Scottish Intercollegiate Guidelines Network. British Guideline on the Management of Asthma. *Thorax* 2003; 58 (Suppl I): S1–S94.
4. Rabe KF, Magnussen H, Dent G. Theophylline and selective PDE inhibitors as bronchodilators and smooth muscle relaxants. *Eur Respir J* 1999; 8: 637–642.
5. Persson CGA, Pauwels, R. Pharmacology of anti-asthma xanthines. In: Page CP, Barnes PJ, eds. *Pharmacology of Asthma*. Berlin: Springer-Verlag, 1991: 207–225.
6. Ziment I. Theophylline and mucociliary clearance. *Chest* 1987; 92 (Suppl 1): 38S–43S.
7. Weinberger M, Hendeles L. Theophylline in asthma. *N Engl J Med* 1996; 334: 1380–1388.
8. Holford N, Black P, Couch R, *et al.* Theophylline target concentration in severe airways obstruction – 10 or 20 mg/litre? A randomised concentration–controlled trial. *Clin Pharmacokinet* 1993; 25: 495–505.
9. Devine BJ. Gentamicin therapy. *Drug Intell Clin Pharm* 1974; 8: 650–655.
10. Traub SL, Johnson CE. Comparison of methods of estimating creatinine clearance in children. *Am J Hosp Pharm* 1980; 37: 195–201.
11. British Medical Association/Royal Pharmaceutical Society of Great Britain. *British National Formulary*, 51. London: BMJ Publishing Group/RPS Publishing, March 2006.
12. Baxter K (ed.). *Stockley's Drug Interactions*, 7th edn. London: Pharmaceutical Press, 2006.

14

Leukotriene receptor antagonists

The story of the leukotriene receptor antagonists (LTRAs) began in 1938, when slow-reacting substance of anaphylaxis (SRS-A) was discovered in the lungs of animals. In 1979, it was discovered that SRS-A was a combination of the leukotrienes LTC4, LTD4 and LTE4, mediators of the asthma response. Further research studies into the leukotriene pathway lead to the development of a new class of anti-asthma therapy, the first for over 20 years. The LTRAs (or anti-leukotrienes) were introduced into clinical practice in the UK in 1997.

Indications

Two LTRAs are licensed in the UK: montelukast and zafirlukast (see Figure 14.1). They are licensed for the treatment of asthma in adults and children (aged 6 months and over for montelukast;[1] aged 12 years and over for zafirlukast[2]). Specifically, montelukast is licensed as add-on therapy for patients with mild-to-moderate asthma that is inadequately controlled by inhaled corticosteroids plus as-required short-acting beta-2 agonists; zafirlukast is licensed for the treatment of asthma. Montelukast is also licensed for the symptomatic treatment of seasonal allergic rhinitis in patients who also have asthma.[1]

Chronic asthma

The current asthma management guideline published by the British Thoracic Society (BTS) and the Scottish Intercollegiate Guidelines Network (SIGN)[3] recommends that LTRAs should be considered as one option at step 3 of the pharmacological management of asthma (see Management Focus, page 217). Specifically, the guideline states that LTRAs should be prescribed only if control of the patient's asthma remains suboptimal despite a trial of long-acting beta-2 agonist, as-required short-acting beta-2 agonist and a high dose of inhaled corticosteroid (e.g. 800 micrograms/day beclometasone or equivalent in adults

Montelukast

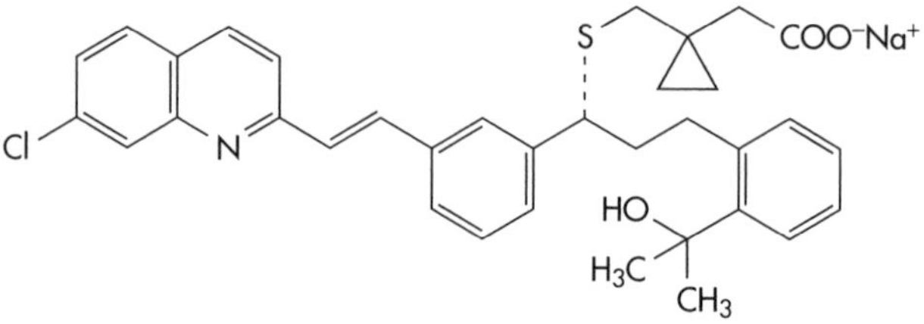

Zafirlukast

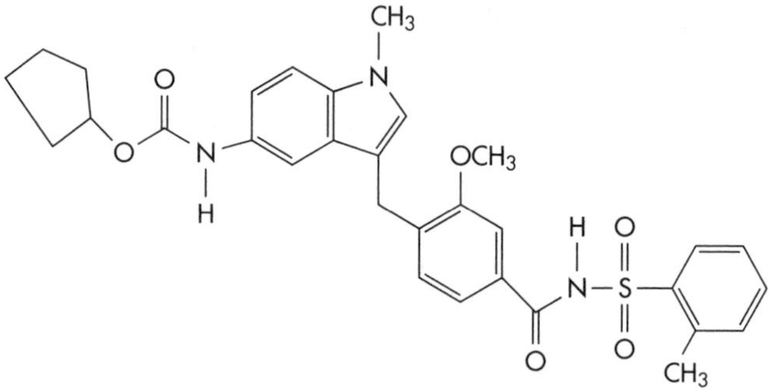

Figure 14.1 Chemical structures of montelukast and zafirlukast.

or 400 micrograms/day in children). This reflects the UK licence for montelukast.

Many clinical studies have investigated the treatment of asthma with an LTRA instead of regular inhaled corticosteroids as first-line therapy to control mild-to-moderate asthma. A meta-analysis of these studies found that corticosteroids were superior in protecting the patient from asthma exacerbations.[4] Patients taking an LTRA were 65% more likely to have an exacerbation requiring oral corticosteroids. The relative risk of an exacerbation, compared with that with inhaled corticosteroids, was similar for montelukast and zafirlukast. Inhaled corticosteroids also improved lung function, symptom scores, daily use of short-acting inhaled beta-2 agonists and quality of life compared with an LTRA.[4] Thus, LTRAs are less effective than inhaled corticosteroids. They can provide additional control when added to inhaled cortico-steroid therapy in patients who are still symptomatic[3] but there is more clinical evidence to support the initial addition of a long-acting beta-2 agonist before an LTRA.[5] Further studies are required to demonstrate whether the LTRAs offer additional benefits for patients who remain symptomatic despite being on inhaled corticosteroids and long-acting beta-2 agonists.

Some clinical studies have shown that the addition of an LTRA may facilitate a reduction in the patient's dose of inhaled corticosteroid whilst maintaining asthma stability. However, a meta-analysis of trials that investigated the corticosteroid-sparing properties of licensed doses of LTRAs concluded that, in patients who were well controlled at baseline, addition of an LTRA did not result in a greater overall reduction in the dose of inhaled corticosteroid compared with placebo, although it was associated with fewer withdrawals because of poorly controlled asthma.[6]

Exercise-induced asthma

Exercise-induced asthma is a common problem for many asthmatics, particularly with the recent emphasis on adequate exercise as part of a healthy lifestyle, and is often an indicator of poor asthma control.

MANAGEMENT FOCUS

Leukotriene receptor antagonists (LTRAs) in the treatment of asthma

---

- LTRAs are not indicated for use in the reversal of bronchospasm in acute asthma attacks.
- Patients should be advised to have appropriate rescue medication available. Therapy with LTRAs can be continued during acute exacerbations of asthma.
- While the dose of inhaled corticosteroids may be reduced gradually under medical supervision, LTRAs should not be abruptly substituted for inhaled or oral corticosteroids. There are no data demonstrating that the dosage of oral corticosteroids can be reduced when montelukast is given concomitantly.
- LTRAs should not be used as monotherapy for the treatment and management of asthma, including exercise-induced asthma.
- As treatment with LTRAs is not effective in all patients, a therapeutic trial for 1 month is usually recommended.
- There appear to be differences between patients in the magnitude of response to LTRAs, but so far it has not been possible to predict which patients will respond best, apart from the rare patients with aspirin-sensitivity asthma, who usually respond.
- Treatment with LTRAs does not negate the need for patients with aspirin-sensitivity asthma to avoid taking aspirin and other non-steroidal anti-inflammatory drugs.

Randomised studies have shown that both montelukast and zafirlukast are effective in inhibiting exercise-induced bronchoconstriction in patients with asthma.[7-9] In adults, montelukast is equivalent to salmeterol in protection against exercise-induced asthma, offering protection for at least 12 hours, making it a good treatment options for athletes whose exertion is prolonged.[8] Whilst the control offered by salmeterol exhibited periodic fluctuations at 4 and 8 weeks, the bronchoprotective effect of montelukast was maintained for 8 weeks with no sign of tolerance.[10]

The prevention and relief of exercise-induced asthma is particularly important in children, for whom physical activity is a large part of everyday life. The daily use of a montelukast 5 mg chewable tablet was superior to placebo in preventing exercise-induced asthma in children aged 6–14 years.[11]

Aspirin-sensitive asthma

A subset of patients with asthma are susceptible to disease exacerbation upon receiving aspirin or other non-steroidal anti-inflammatory drugs (NSAIDs). This clinical syndrome, called aspirin-sensitive asthma (ASA), is associated with alterations in arachidonic acid metabolism and oversynthesis of the cysteinyl leukotrienes (see Figure 2.4, page 17). The addition of an LTRA for adults with ASA/NSAID-sensitive asthma that is inadequately controlled on inhaled corticosteroids improves control of symptoms.[12] In patients with ASA already requiring moderate-to-high doses of inhaled corticosteroids, montelukast provides additional improvements in lung function, requirement for rescue medication, sleep quality and asthma-specific quality-of-life scores, and reduces exacerbations. Montelukast also improved nasal symptoms in patients with chronic nasal symptoms associated with ASA.[13]

Atopic disorders

Leukotrienes are important pro-inflammatory mediators in allergic rhinitis and eczema. Currently montelukast (10 mg) is the only LTRA licensed for the treatment of seasonal allergic rhinitis in patients who also have asthma. Although allergic rhinitis is not a life-threatening condition, the clinical symptoms – nasal congestion and itching, rhinorrhoea, sneezing and nasal pruritus – can significantly disrupt a patient's quality of life.[14] Clinical studies have highlighted that more complete control of these symptoms is achieved with a combination of an antihistamine with an LTRA than either agent alone or placebo.[15]

Mechanism of action

The leukotrienes (LTC4, LTD4 and LTE4) are metabolites of arachidonic acid formed by the 5-lipoxygenase pathway (see Figure 2.4, page 17) and are inflammatory mediators released by inflammatory cells, particularly mast cells, neutrophils, eosinophils and macrophages.[16,17] The effects of the leukotrienes are mediated mainly through the cys-LT1 receptor, found in the human airway. Leukotriene-mediated effects in asthma include airway oedema, microvascular leakage, smooth muscle contraction, mucus secretion and recruitment of eosinophils into the airway. Leukotrienes may also be involved in airway remodelling in asthma, causing hyperplasia of bronchial smooth muscle and airway epithelium. They have an important pathophysiological role in asthma and rhinitis and are involved in both the early and late asthmatic responses to allergen challenge. Leukotrienes can be detected in bronchoalveolar lavage fluid and in the urine of patients with asthma during an exacerbation or allergen challenge. Release of leukotrienes is increased during an acute asthma attack and falls as the attack resolves; levels are particularly high in people with ASA.

Both montelukast and zafirlukast are orally active compounds that bind with high affinity and selectivity to the cys-LT1 receptor. They work by preventing leukotrienes from binding to the cys-LT1 receptors, thereby preventing the physiological actions of leukotrienes. LTRAs also have mild anti-inflammatory effects and may reduce the eosinophilic inflammation provoked by the leukotrienes.[16]

Pharmacokinetics

Montelukast[1]

Montelukast is rapidly absorbed following oral administration. The mean oral bioavailability is 64%. After administration of the 10 mg film-coated tablet to fasted adults, the mean peak plasma concentration is achieved in 3–4 hours; bronchodilation occurs about 2 hours after administration and the duration of action is about 24 hours, enabling once-daily dosing. Montelukast is more than 99% bound to plasma proteins and has a steady-state volume of distribution of 8–11 litres. It is extensively metabolised in the liver by cytochrome P450 isoenzymes CYP3A4 and CYP2C9. Therapeutic plasma concentrations of montelukast do not inhibit these cytochromes and there are minimal drug–drug interactions.

Montelukast and its metabolites are excreted almost exclusively via the bile. In several studies, the mean plasma half-life of montelukast ranged from 2.7 to 5.5 hours in healthy young adults. No dosage adjustment is required in the elderly or in patients with mild-to-moderate hepatic insufficiency or renal insufficiency.

Zafirlukast[2]

Zafirlukast is rapidly absorbed following oral administration. Administration of zafirlukast with food reduces the mean bioavailability by approximately 40%, so it should be taken 1 hour before or 2 hours after food. Peak plasma concentrations are generally achieved 3 hours after oral administration and the duration of action is about 12 hours. Zafirlukast is more than 99% bound to plasma proteins and has a steady-state volume of distribution of approximately 70 litres, suggesting moderate distribution into tissues. It is extensively metabolised by cytochrome P450 isoenzyme CYP2C9 to significantly more active metabolites. Therapeutic plasma concentrations of zafirlukast inhibit isoenzymes CYP3A4 and CYP2C9, resulting in a number of drug–drug interactions (discussed below). Biliary excretion is the primary route of excretion. The mean plasma half-life is 8–16 hours.

The manufacturer advises prescribing with caution in patients with moderate-to-severe renal impairment and to avoid using zafirlukast in patients with hepatic insufficiency. Clinical experience with zafirlukast in the elderly (over 65 years) is limited and caution is recommended until further information is available.

Dosage

The recommended dosages of the LTRAs are summarised in Table 14.1.

Contraindications

Both montelukast and zafirlukast are contraindicated in patients with known hypersensitivity to the active substances or to any of the excipients.[1,2] Zafirlukast is also contraindicated in patients with hepatic impairment or cirrhosis and in children under 12 years of age.[2]

Adverse effects

LTRAs are generally well tolerated. Common adverse effects include headache, nausea and vomiting, gastrointestinal disturbances, skin rashes and occasional abnormalities of liver function tests.[1,2] Zafirlukast

Table 14.1 Summary of the dosages and indications for the leukotriene receptor antagonists

Leukotriene receptor antagonist	Recommended dosage	Indication and comments
Montelukast (Singulair; MSD)	Adults and children over 15 years and older: 10 mg at night Children aged 6–14 years: paediatric tablets, 5 mg at night Children aged 6 months–5 years: paediatric granules 4 mg (one sachet) at night	Add-on therapy for patients with mild-to-moderate asthma that is inadequately controlled by inhaled corticosteroids plus as-needed short-acting beta-2 agonists The 10 mg tablet is licensed for adults with asthma and concomitant seasonal allergic rhinitis
Zafirlukast (Accolate, AstraZeneca)	Adults and children aged 12 years and above: 20 mg twice daily Not recommended for children under 12 years	Prophylaxis of asthma Food may reduce the bioavailability of zafirlukast so the tablets should not be taken with food

can produce liver abnormalities, so it is important to do liver function tests[2] (see Adverse Effects Focus, below). Montelukast has been associated with psychiatric and behavioural disorders, nightmares and other sleep disorders.[1]

Churg–Strauss syndrome

A few cases of Churg–Strauss syndrome have been observed following LTRA administration. Churg–Strauss syndrome is a rare but often fatal multisystem allergic granulomatous vasculitis affecting small and medium-sized arteries. It mostly affects the lungs and may itself trigger asthma. Patients often present with influenza-like symptoms, such as fever, myalgia, headache and weight loss. Other systemic signs include eosinophilia, vasculitic rash, cardiac complications (such as heart failure, myocarditis, pericarditis and myocardial infarction), gastro-intestinal symptoms (abdominal pain, diarrhoea, gastrointestinal

ADVERSE EFFECTS FOCUS

Zafirlukast-induced hepatotoxicity

- Cases of life-threatening hepatic failure have been reported in patients treated with zafirlukast. Cases of liver injury with no other associated cause have been reported in post-marketing adverse-event surveillance of patients who have received the recommended dose of zafirlukast (40 mg/day). In the majority of cases, the patient's symptoms improved and their liver enzymes returned to normal or near normal after stopping zafirlukast. In rare cases, patients have either presented with fulminant hepatitis or have progressed to hepatic failure and death.
- Periodic testing of liver function has not been proven to prevent serious injury but it is generally believed that early detection of drug-induced hepatic injury, along with immediate withdrawal of the suspect drug enhances the likelihood of recovery.
- Patients should be advised to be alert for signs and symptoms of liver dysfunction, (e.g. right-upper quadrant pain, nausea, fatigue, lethargy, pruritus, jaundice, flu-like symptoms, anorexia and enlarged liver) and to contact their doctor immediately if they occur.
- If liver dysfunction is suspected, zafirlukast should be discontinued immediately. Liver function tests should be measured and the patient managed accordingly.
- Patients in whom zafirlukast is withdrawn because of hepatic dysfunction where no other cause is found should not be re-exposed to zafirlukast.

bleeding) and peripheral neuropathy. The majority of cases can be treated effectively with oral corticosteroids and more severe cases are treated with immunosuppressive agents such as cyclophosphamide. Incidences of Churg-Strauss syndrome following an LTRA have usually, but not always, been associated with a reduction of oral corticosteroid therapy. There has been some speculation that the syndrome is an existing condition in these patients that was masked by the corticosteroid and was revealed when the steroid dose was reduced and hence may not be a side-effect of the drug. Hence, patients taking an LTRA should not stop taking or change the dose of other asthma medications unless instructed to do so by their doctor. Although in clinical trials some patients were able to maintain asthma control with lower doses of inhaled corticosteroids, the LTRAs should not be substituted for inhaled or oral corticosteroids.

Drug interactions

Montelukast[1]

In drug-interaction studies, the recommended clinical dose of montelukast did not have clinically important effects on the pharmacokinetics of the following drugs: theophylline, prednisolone, fexofenadine, oral contraceptives (norethindrone 1 mg/ethinylestradiol 35 micrograms), digoxin and warfarin. Since montelukast is metabolised by the cytochrome P450 isoenzyme CYP3A4, caution should be taken when administered in conjunction with inducers of this enzyme, such as phenytoin, phenobarbital and rifampicin, but no dosage adjustment is recommended.

Zafirlukast[2]

Rare incidences of increases in theophylline levels, with or without clinical signs or symptoms of theophylline toxicity, have been observed after the addition of zafirlukast to an existing theophylline regimen. The mechanism of this interaction is unknown and further studies are required. No dosage adjustment is recommended, although it would seem sensible to monitor the effects of concurrent use.

Co-administration of zafirlukast with warfarin results in a clinically significant increase in prothrombin time. Patients taking warfarin and zafirlukast should therefore have their prothrombin times monitored closely and the dose of warfarin adjusted accordingly. This interaction is probably due to inhibition of cytochrome P450 isoenzyme CYP2C9 by zafirlukast. Care should be exercised when administering zafirlukast with other drugs metabolised by CYP2C9, such as phenytoin, carbamazepine and tolbutamide. Erythromycin may decrease the bioavailability of zafirlukast, leading to a reduction in plasma zafirlukast levels and possibly a reduced response.

Preparations

An advantage of the LTRAs is that they are formulated as oral tablets. Long-term concordance is therefore likely to be better with this therapy than with the use of inhaled preparations. The preparations of the LTRAs are summarised in Table 14.1.

References

1. Merck Sharp & Dohme Ltd. Singulair 10 mg tablets/4 and 5 mg paediatric tablets. *Summary of product characteristics*. May 2006.
2. AstraZeneca UK Ltd. Accolate. *Summary of product characteristics*. December 2004.
3. British Thoracic Society/Scottish Intercollegiate Guidelines Network. British Guideline on the Management of Asthma. *Thorax* 2003; 58 (Suppl I): S1–S94.
4. Duchame FM, Di Salvio. Anti-leukotrienes compared to inhaled corticosteroids in the management of recurrent and/or chronic asthma in adults and children. *The Cochrane Library*, issue 1. Chichester: John Wiley & Sons, 2004 (www.thecochranelibrary.com).
5. Ram FSF, Cates CJ, Ducharme FM. Long-acting beta2-agonists versus antileukotrienes as add-on therapy to inhaled corticosteroids for chronic asthma. *The Cochrane Library*, issue 1. Chichester: John Wiley & Sons, 2005 (www.thecochranelibrary.com).
6. Ducharme F, Schwartz Z, Kakuma R. Addition of anti-leukotriene agents to inhaled corticosteroids for chronic asthma. *The Cochrane Library*, issue 1. Chichester: John Wiley & Sons, 2004 (www.thecochranelibrary.com).
7. Leff JA, Busse WW, Pearlman D, *et al*. Montelukast, a leukotriene-receptor antagonist, for the treatment of mild asthma and exercise-induced bronchoconstriction. *N Engl J Med* 1998; 399: 147–152.
8. Coreno A, Skowronski M, Kotaru C, *et al*. Comparative effects of long-acting beta-2-agonists, leukotriene receptor antagonists, and a 5-lipoxygenase inhibitor on exercise-induced asthma. *J Allergy Clin Immunol* 2000; 106: 500–506.
9. Dessanges JR, Prefaut C, Taytard A, *et al*. The effect of zafirlukast on repetitive exercise-induced bronchoconstriction: the possible role of leukotrienes in exercise-induced refractoriness. *J Allergy Clin Immunol* 1999; 104: 1155–1161.

10. Edelman JM, Turpin JA, Bronsky EA, *et al.* Oral Montelukast compared with inhaled salmeterol to prevent exercise-induced bronchoconstriction: A randomised, double blind trial. *Ann Intern Med* 2000; 132: 97–104.

11. Kemp J, Dockhorn R, Shapiro G, *et al.* Montelukast once daily inhibits exercise-induced bronchoconstriction in 6–14-year-old children with asthma. *J Pediatr* 1998; 133: 424–428.

12. Dahlen SE, Malmstrom K, Nizankowska E, *et al.* Improvement of aspirin-intolerant asthma by montelukast, a leukotriene antagonist. A randomized, double-blind, placebo-controlled trial. *Am J Respir Crit Care Med* 2002; 165: 9–14.

13. Micheletto C, Tognella S, Visconti M, *et al.* Montelukast 10mg improves nasal function and nasal response to aspirin in ASA-sensitive asthmatics: a controlled study vs placebo. *Allergy* 2004; 59: 289–294.

14. Bousquet J, Duchateau J, Pignat JC, *et al.* Improvement of quality of life by treatment with cetirizine in patients with perennial allergic rhinitis as determined by a French version of the SF-36 questionnaire. *J Allergy Clin Immunol* 1996; 98: 309–316.

15. Kurowski M, Kuna P, Gorski P. Montelukast plus cetirizine in the prophylactic treatment of seasonal allergic rhinitis: influence on clinical symptoms and nasal allergic inflammation. *Allergy* 2004; 59: 280–288.

16. Barnes NC, Kuitert LM. Drugs affecting the leukotriene pathway in asthma. *Br J Clin Prac* 1995; 49: 262–266.

17. Busse W, Kraft M. Cysteinyl leukotrienes in allergic inflammation. *Chest* 2005; 127: 1312–1326.

15

New therapies and future developments in asthma management

The only new class of drug developed for the treatment of asthma in the last 30 years have been the leukotriene receptor antagonists. It has proved difficult to develop new anti-asthma drugs, partly because the existing drugs, especially the inhaled corticosteroids and beta-2 agonists, are so effective. There is, however, a need for even more effective therapies that reduce airway inflammatory processes, achieve effective bronchodilation of the airways and reduce the airway remodelling processes.

Improved understanding of asthma has led to the development of several new treatments for asthma. One agent licensed in 2005 for the management of atopic asthma is omalizumab, an anti-immunoglobulin E (IgE) monoclonal antibody described in more detail below. Other agents being tested in clinical trials include selective phosphodiesterase (PDE) inhibitors, mediator antagonists and adhesion molecules.

Omalizumab

The formation of circulating IgE antibodies to allergens appears to be crucial in the sequence of cellular events that leads to an allergic reaction such as that which occurs in asthma and allergic rhinitis. The exposure to allergens (such as house dust mite) leads to an IgE-dependent activation and release of key inflammatory mediators, including histamine, prostaglandins and leukotrienes from mast cells and basophils. Various strategies have been investigated in attempts to reduce this interaction but it has proved difficult to achieve. An alternative approach is to decrease the levels of circulating IgE available to interact with the mediator or effector cells. This rationale is supported by evidence that serum levels of IgE correlate with the severity of asthma symptoms. Omalizumab is a highly specific monoclonal antibody that binds to circulating IgE and prevents receptor binding on effector cells (see Figure 15.1).

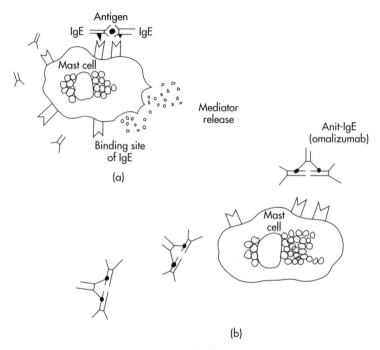

Figure 15.1 The mechanism of action of the monoclonal antibody omalizumab. Immunoglobulin E (IgE) molecules bind to high-affinity binding sites on the surface of mast cells and basophils, and to anti-IgE. **(a)** Cross linkage of IgE by allergens on the cell surface causes the release of inflammatory mediators. **(b)** Anti-IgE binds to the portion of IgE that recognises the receptor on the surface of mast cells and basophils. This prevents the immunoglobulin from binding to and activating these cells. The number of receptors also decreases. (From: Chung FK. Omalizumab: IgE antibody for difficult-to-treat asthma. *Future Prescriber* 2001; 2(6); 13, reproduced with permission of Wiley Interface Ltd.)

Since the discovery of the anti-IgE strategy 8 years ago, the safety and efficacy of omalizumab in patients with allergic asthma and rhinitis have been evaluated in a number of randomised, double-blind, placebo-controlled, multicentre trials.[1-5] In these trials, patients had had asthma for at least one year and required treatment with inhaled corticosteroids. All patients had at least one positive skin-prick test to a perennial aero-allergen (specifically, dust mites, cockroaches or dog or cat dander), as well as an elevated total serum IgE level. During the course of each trial, inhaled corticosteroids were initially maintained at a stable dose, followed by a phase of dose reduction to the lowest dose required for asthma control. The data have shown that omalizumab reduces the rate of asthma exacerbations and visits to hospital emergency departments in patients with inadequately controlled asthma. Omalizumab has also been shown to reduce patients' overall dose of inhaled corticosteroids[6] and improves patients' asthma-related quality of life.[7] Further work with omalizumab demonstrated that it has important benefits in patients with poorly controlled asthma despite high-dose inhaled corticosteroid therapy,[8] and analysis of clinical data suggests that the patients who respond best to anti-IgE therapy are those with asthma at the more severe end of the spectrum.[9]

The place of omalizumab in the management of asthma has not yet been clearly defined. The following patients are particularly likely to benefit from the use of omalizumab:

- patients with evidence of sensitisation to perennial aeroallergens
- patients on high doses of inhaled cortisoteroids that have a potential risk of adverse effects
- patients with frequent exacerbations of asthma.

Analysis of pooled data from published trials has indicated that patients who responded to omalizumab had a forced expiratory volume in 1 second (FEV_1) of less than 65% predicted, were taking doses of inhaled corticosteroids equivalent to more than 800 micrograms beclometasone per day, and had been admitted to hospital at least once in the past year. Patients requiring a maintenance dose of oral corticosteroid to control their asthma may be less likely to respond to omalizumab.[9,10]

Omalizumab offers a number of advantages for patients with moderate-to-severe asthma. These include:

- reducing the number of exacerbations
- targeting the allergic component of asthma for the first time
- reducing the dosage of inhaled or oral corticosteroids and therefore the risks of adverse effects
- the opportunity to control concordance with prescribed medication, as injections will initially be given by a health professional.

The dose and frequency of injection of omalizumab are determined by total serum IgE levels, which are measured before the start of treatment, and body weight. Total serum IgE levels should be between 30 and 700 IU/mL (for patients aged 12–75 years). Monitoring of total serum IgE levels during treatment with omalizumab is not indicated because levels will be elevated by the presence of circulating IgE–anti-IgE complexes. Doses range from 150 to 375 mg, administered subcutaneously every 2–4 weeks. Omalizumab is supplied as a lyophilised sterile powder in single use vials, which must be stored at temperatures of 2–8°C. The injection takes 10–20 minutes or more to reconstitute with sterile water and must not be shaken, as this may inactivate the drug. Once prepared, the drug must be used within 4 hours if at room temperature or 8 hours if refrigerated. These requirements plus the high cost of the drug mean that many clinics are organised so that the drug is not prepared until the patient arrives. This results in visits that take an hour or more, as 30 minutes' observation after the injection is recommended.

It can take several weeks for a response to omalizumab to become apparent; a trial period of 16 weeks is therefore recommended. In a clinical trial, 87% of patients who responded to omalizumab by 16 weeks had done so by 12 weeks.[9]

Potential safety concerns identified from the trial data on omalizumab included risks of developing cancer or anaphylaxis. Cancer developed in more patients treated with omalizumab then those who received placebo; omalizumab is therefore not currently recommended for patients with a history of cancer or strong family history of cancer until this risk is better understood. Other adverse effects included rash, diarrhoea, nausea, vomiting, menorrhagia, haematoma and injection-site reactions.

The efficacy and safety of omalizumab beyond 1 year have not been established. Since asthma is a chronic disease, however, studies are needed to evaluate long-term efficacy and safety.

Omalizumab represents a new approach in the treatment of asthma. However, production of the monoclonal antibodies is expensive. Omalizumab is considerably more expensive than conventional asthma therapy and the likely cost-effectiveness of this treatment must be assessed before prescribing. The manufacturer estimates that usage could be about 33 patients per 100 000 population over 5 years. Although this is likely to have a significant impact on prescribing budgets, the costs associated with hospitalisations and corticosteroid use will be reduced, which may make it economically as well as clinically attractive. The asthma management guideline published by the British Thoracic Society (BTS) and the Scottish Intercollegiate Guidelines Network (SIGN) suggests that omalizumab may be of benefit in selected patients with severe persistent allergic asthma, but at present its role in the stepwise management of asthma is unclear.[10]

The National Institute for Health and Clinical Excellence (NICE) expects to publish guidance on the use of omalizumab in asthma in February 2008.

Selective phosphodiesterase inhibitors

Beta-2 agonist bronchodilators act by increasing levels of intracellular cyclic 3,5-adenosine monophosphate (cAMP) and reducing intracellular calcium ion concentration, leading to dilatation of airway smooth muscle (see Chapter 10). The cAMP is metabolised and inactivated by the PDE enzymes. PDE inhibitors therefore increase cAMP levels, leading to relaxation of smooth muscle, working synergistically with beta-2 agonists. The principal action of the methylxanthines is likely to be non-selective inhibition of PDE activity (see Chapter 13). The major PDEs within bronchial smooth muscle are types 3 and 4 and selective inhibitors of PDE3 and PDE4 are currently being developed. Roflumilast, an orally active PDE4 inhibitor, is in late phase III clinical development. The effectiveness and safety profile of therapeutic selective PDE3 and PDE4 inhibitors await evaluation but it is hoped that they will be more effective than theophylline and will not share its adverse effects.

Mediator antagonists

Many different inflammatory mediators have now been implicated in asthma. Antagonism of one or several of these mediators may improve asthma management, and several potential therapeutic agents are currently being investigated (see Table 15.1). As many mediators probably contribute to the pathological features of asthma, it seems unlikely that a single antagonist will have a major clinical effect compared with non-specific agents such as beta-2 agonists and corticosteroids. Results of trials in asthmatic patients have been disappointing, despite promising results in animal models. The only class of mediator antagonist to show useful clinical effect to date are the leukotriene receptor antagonists (see Chapter 14).

Anti-interleukin-4 and -5 therapies[11]

Interleukin (IL)-4 has a broad range of biological effects. In general terms it can be described as the main cytokine involved in the pathogenesis of allergic responses. Production of IgE following contact with an allergen depends on cytokine IL-4 (and/or IL-13). IgE-mediated immune responses are further enhanced by IL-4 through its ability to upregulate IgE receptors on the cell surface. IL-4 also stimulates mucus-producing cells and fibroblasts and therefore appears to be involved in

Table 15.1 Inhibitors of inflammatory mediators and cytokines

Mediator	Examples of inhibitors
Inflammatory mediators	
Histamine	Acrivastine, cetirizine, chlorphenamine, fexofenadine, loratadine
Leukotriene D4	Zafirlukast, montelukast, zileuton
Leukotriene B4	LY 293111
Platelet activating factor	Apafant, modipafent, bepafant
Thromboxane	Ozagrel
Bradykinin	Icatibant
Adenosine	Theophylline
Nitric oxide	Aminoguanidine
Reactive oxygen species	N-acetylcysteine, ascorbic acid
Endothelin	Bosentan
Cytokines	
IL-4	IL-4 antibody, soluble IL-4 receptor
IL-5	IL-5 antibody (SCH55700, mepolizumab)
Anti-TNF-alpha	Etanercept

IL, interleukin; TNF, tumour necrosis factor.

the airway remodelling process. Inhalation of recombinant human IL-4 induces airway eosinophilia and causes airway hyperresponsiveness in atopic asthmatics. Antibodies to IL-4 have been used to block production of IgE *in vitro* and *in vivo*. When administered to mice, anti-IL-4 antibodies can prevent the induction of an IgE response to the sensitising antigen.[12] Another promising approach to inhibiting the effects of IL-4 is the production of a soluble IL-4 receptor (IL-4R), which is capable of interacting with IL-4 even though it lacks the transmembrane and cytoplasmic domains. It does not induce cellular activation but instead binds and neutralises circulating cytokines.

In preliminary investigations, IL-4R proved safe and effective in the treatment of patients with asthma.[13,14] In a phase I study, subjects with mild or moderate persistent asthma were withdrawn from their inhaled corticosteroids and randomly assigned to receive placebo or IL-4R, 0.5 or 1.5 mg by nebuliser. There were no significant adverse events related to the study drug and no patients developed antibodies against

IL-4R. Pharmacokinetic analysis demonstrated a prolonged serum half-life of about 5 days, suggesting that weekly therapy would be effective. Treatment with IL-4R, 1.5 mg, was associated with significantly better FEV_1, asthma symptom score, quality-of-life scores and beta-2-agonist use.[13] In a phase I/II double-blind, placebo-controlled study, 62 patients with moderate persistent asthma were randomised to 12-weekly IL-4R, 0.75, 1.5 or 3.0 mg or placebo by nebuliser. FEV_1 decreased dramatically in the placebo group but not the 3.0 mg treatment group over the 3-month treatment period.[14]

IL-5 promotes eosinophil mobilisation within the airway. In asthma, there is an increase in IL-5 production, and it is known that increased serum IL-5 is associated with a fall in the FEV_1. Hence, it is logical to think that a monoclonal antibody to IL-5 could be of benefit in asthma. Humanised monoclonal antibodies to IL-5 have been developed, and a single intravenous infusion markedly reduces blood eosinophils for several weeks and prevents eosinophil recruitment in to the airways after allergen challenge in patients with mild asthma. However, this treatment has no significant effect on the early or late response to allergen challenge, baseline hyperreactivity or airway hyper-responsiveness to histamine.[15]

Anti-tumour necrosis factor-alpha

Tumour necrosis factor (TNF) is released in allergic responses from mast cells and macrophages via IgE-dependent mechanisms. TNF-alpha is expressed in the airways of asthmatics and may play an important role in increasing inflammation within the lung.[16–20] Drugs that target TNF-alpha have been developed to neutralise the detrimental effects of this inflammatory cytokine and have proved to be safe and effective in the treatment of patients with rheumatoid arthritis, Crohn's disease or psoriasis refractory to conventional treatments. Biological therapies that block TNF-alpha are likely to represent a considerable advance in the management of patients with difficult asthma that is particularly resistant to typical treatment modalities.

The two strategies for inhibiting TNF-alpha that have been most extensively studied to date consist of monoclonal anti-TNF-alpha antibodies and soluble TNF-alpha receptors (sTNF-R). Both will theoretically bind to circulating TNF-alpha, thus limiting its ability to engage with cell-membrane-bound TNF receptors and activate inflammatory pathways. The best studied of the monoclonal anti-TNF-alpha antibodies is infliximab. Etanercept is the best studied of the anti-sTNF-R and is approved for the treatment of rheumatoid arthritis in adults and in children. A recent study in patients with mild asthma reported a significant improvement in symptoms and lung function following treatment with anti-TNF.[19] A further study showed that the administration of etanercept to patients with severe asthma was associated with improvement in asthma symptoms, lung function and bronchial hyperresponsiveness.[20] The effects of anti-TNF therapy in asthma now require confirmation in placebo-controlled studies.

Anti-adhesion therapies

Adhesion receptors located in airway membranes are involved in many aspects of the immune response. Agents that block the action of these receptors have the potential to be potent anti-inflammatory drugs.[21] While blocking adhesion molecules is an exciting approach to asthma treatment, there may be potential dangers in inhibiting immune responses, leading to increased numbers of infections and increased risk of neoplasia. Further studies are required.

Eosinophils and asthma management

Asthma is generally managed by evaluating patients' symptoms and their use of relief medication, and monitoring simple measures of lung function, according to the BTS/SIGN asthma management guideline[22] (see Chapters 3 and 6).

Eosinophils are thought to have an important pro-inflammatory role in the pathogenesis of asthma,[23] and that suppression with corticosteroids is usually associated with improvements in symptoms and airway function. A new approach being investigated in the management of asthma involves using the patient's induced sputum eosinophil count to guide treatment. Anti-inflammatory treatment, usually inhaled corticosteroids, is increased if the sputum eosinophil count rises above a cut-off point of 3%; it is kept the same dose if the count is between 1 and 3%, and it is reduced if it is below 1%. This is done irrespective of asthma control. This technique has been shown to significantly reduce asthma exacerbations with fewer rescue courses of oral corticosteroids. Symptom scores, peak expiratory flow, use of rescue beta-2 agonists and all other drugs were shown to be similar when compared with a group of patients with asthma managed according to the BTS/SIGN asthma management guideline.[24] Patients who had low sputum eosinophil counts received fewer inhaled corticosteroids than patients managed according to the standard guideline. Normalising the induced sputum eosinophil count may therefore be a novel approach to managing patients with severe asthma who are not responding to standard management. Further work is required before the findings of controlled studies are extrapolated into routine clinical practice.

Single inhaled therapy

There is now compelling evidence that, compared with using an inhaled corticosteroid alone, the addition of a long-acting inhaled beta-2 agonist to an inhaled corticosteroid improves control of asthma in terms of reduced symptoms, improved lung function and fewer exacerbation in patients with mild, moderate or persistent asthma.[25] This led to the development of fixed-combination inhalers – salmeterol plus fluticasone, and formoterol plus budesonide – which are being used increasingly in asthma management. It is normal practice to administer these combination inhalers twice daily at a dose that is related to the severity of asthma, and to use a short-acting beta-2 agonist as required to relieve any breakthrough symptoms. Frequent use of the short-acting beta-2 agonist indicates poor control and the need for a higher maintenance dose of the combination inhaler or poor compliance with the inhaler.

The long-acting beta-2 agonist formoterol has also been shown to be effective as a reliever medication in asthma, as it has a rapid onset of action with a long bronchodilator effect, but with similar systemic side-effects as the short-acting beta-2 agonists.[26] A new approach in the management of asthma is the prescribing of just a formoterol/budesonide combination inhaler (i.e. no short-acting beta-2 agonist). Patients are told to use the combination inhaler twice a day and to take additional puffs as needed for symptom control. Clinical trials have shown that this novel approach reduces the number of severe asthma exacerbations, reduces the need for oral corticosteroids and improves symptom control and lung function compared with the standard treatment regimen.[27–31] However, one concern about this approach is that some patients might end up using the combination inhaler frequently and therefore receive an unacceptably high dose of inhaled corticosteroid, although this was not the case in a 1 year study, the mean number of additional doses being only one per day.[31]

The prescribing of a single inhaler for both maintenance and rescue of asthma symptoms will help to simplify asthma therapy for patients and health professionals and is likely to improve compliance. It also follows what patients do in the real world, where they tend to take more medication in response to worsening symptoms. However, effectiveness studies in routine clinical practice are required to see whether this simplified approach is applicable to treating asthma patients in the community.

References

1. Buhl R, Soler M, Matz J, et al. Omalizumab provides long-term control in patients with moderate to severe allergic asthma. *J Eur Respir* 2002; 20: 73–78.
2. Holgate ST, Chuchalin AG, Hebert J, et al. Efficacy and safety of a recombinant anti-immunoglobulin E antibody (omalizumab) in severe allergic asthma. *Clin Exp Allergy* 2004; 34: 632–638.
3. Holgate S, Bousquet J, Wenzel S, et al. Efficacy of omalizumab and anti-immunoglobulin E antibody in patients with allergic asthma at high risk of serious asthma-related morbidity and mortality. *Curr Med Res Opin* 2001; 17: 233–240.
4. Vignola AM, Humbert M, Bousquet J, et al. Efficacy and tolerability of anti-immunoglobulin E therapy with omalizumab in patients with concomitant allergic asthma and persistent allergic rhinitis: SOLAR. *Allergy* 2004; 59: 709–717.
5. Busse W, Corren J, Lanier BQ, et al. Omalizumab, anti-IgE recombinant humanised monocloncal antibody, for the treatment of severe allergic asthma. *J Allergy Clin Immunol* 2001; 108: 184–190.
6. Soler M, Matz J, Townley R, et al. The anti-IgE antibody omalizumab reduces exacerbations and steroid requirements in allergic asthmatics. *Eur Respir J* 2001; 18: 254–261.
7. Buhl R, Hant G, Solèr M, et al. The anti-IgE antibody omalizumab improves asthma-related quality of life in patients with allergic asthma. *Eur Respir J* 2002; 20: 1088–1094.
8. Humbert M, Beasley R, Ayres J, et al. Benefits of omalizumab as add-on therapy in patients with severe persistent asthma who are inadequately controlled despite best available therapy (GINA 2002 step 4 treatment): INNOVATE. *Allergy* 2005; 60: 309–316.
9. Bousquet J, Cabrera P, Berkman N, et al. The effect of treatment with omalizumab, an anti-IgE antibody, on asthma exacerbations and emergency medical visits in patients with severe persistent asthma. *Allergy* 2005; 60: 302–308.
10. British Thoracic Society/Scottish Intercollegiate Guidelines Network. *British Guideline on the Management of Asthma*. Revised November 2005. www.enterpriseportal2.co.uk/filestore/bts/asthmaupdatenov05.pdf
11. Zhou CY, Crocker IC, Koenig G, et al. Anti-interleukin-4 inhibits immunoglobulin E production in a murine model of atopic asthma. *J Asthma* 1997; 34:195–201.
12. Borish L, Nelson H, Lanz M, et al. Recombinant human interleukin-4 receptor in moderate astopic asthma: a randomized double-blind, placebo-controlled pilot study. *Am J Respir Crit Care Med* 1999; 160: 1816–1823.
13. Borish L, Nelson H, Corren J, et al. Phase I/II study of recombinant

interleukin-4 receptor (IL-4R) in adult patients with moderate asthma. *J Allergy Clin Immunol* 2000; 105: A828.

14. Leckie MJ, Brinke A, Khan J, *et al*. Effects of an interleukin-5 blocking monoclonal antibody on eosinophils, airway hyper-responsiveness, and the late asthmatic response. *Lancet* 2001; 356: 2144–2148.

15. Kips JC, Tournoy KG, Pauwels RA. New anti-asthma therapies: suppression of the effect of interleukin (IL-4) and IL-5. *Eur Respir J* 2001; 17: 499–506.

16. Kips JC, Tavernier J, Pauwels RA. Tumour necrosis factor causes bronchial hyperresponsiveness in rats. *Am Rev Respir Dis* 1992; 145: 332–336.

17. Thomas PS, Yates DH, Barnes PJ. Tumour necrosis factor-alpha increases airway responsiveness and sputum neutrophilia in normal human subjects. *Am J Respir Crit Care Med* 1995; 152: 76–80.

18. Thomas PS. Tumour necrosis factor-alpha: the role of this multifunctional cytokine in asthma. *Immunol Cell Biol* 2001; 79: 132–140.

19. Thomas PS, Heywood G. Effects of inhaled tumour necrosis factor alpha in subjects with mild asthma. *Thorax* 2002; 57: 774–778.

20. Howarth PH, Babu KS, Arshad HS, *et al*. Tumour necrosis factor (TNF-alpha) as a novel therapeutic target in symptomatic corticosteroid dependent asthma. *Thorax* 2005; 60: 1012–1018.

21. Ulbrich H, Eriksson EE, Lindbom L. Leukocyte and endothelial cell adhesion molecules as targets for therapeutic interventions in inflammatory disease. *Trends Pharmacol Sci* 2003; 24: 640–647.

22. British Thoracic Society/Scottish Intercollegiate Guidelines Network. British Guideline on the Management of Asthma. *Thorax* 2003; 58 (Suppl I): S1–S94.

23. Wardlaw AJ, Brightling C, Green R, *et al*. Eosinophils in asthma and other allergic diseases. *Br Med Bull* 2000: 56: 985–1003.

24. Green RH, Brightling CE, McKenna S, *et al*. Asthma exacerbations and sputum eosinophil counts: a randomised controlled trial. *Lancet* 2002; 360: 1715–1721.

25. Walters EH, Walters JA, Gibson MD. Inhaled long acting beta-2 agonists for stable chronic asthma. *The Cochrane Library*, issue 4. Chichester: John Wiley & Sons, 2003 (*www.thecochranelibrary.com*).

26. Tattersfield AE, Lofdahl CG, Postma DS, *et al*. Comparison of formoterol and terbutaline for as-needed treatment of asthma: a randomised trial. *Lancet* 2001; 357: 257–261.

27. Vogelmeier C, D'Urzo A, Jaspal M, *et al*. Symbicort for both maintenance and relief reduces exacerbations compared with a titration of seretide (Advair) in patients with asthma: a real-life study. Abstract presented at the 102nd American Thoracic Society International Conference, San Diego, USA, May 2005.

28. D'Urzo A, Vogelmeier C, Jaspal M, *et al*. Symbicort (budesonide/formoterol) for both maintenance and relief reduces the exacerbation burden compared with a titration of seretide (salmeterol/fluticasone) in patients with asthma: a real-life study. Abstract presented at the 102nd American Thoracic Society International Conference, San Diego, USA, May, 2005.

29. Rabe KF, Pizzichini E, Ställberg B, *et al*. Single inhaler therapy with budesonide/formoterol provides superior asthma control compared with fixed dosing with budesonide plus terbutaline as needed. Abstract presented at the

60th International Meeting of the American Academy of Allergy, Asthma and Immunology (AAAAI), San Francisco, USA, March, 2004.

30. Scicchitano R, Aalbers R, Ukena D, *et al*. Efficacy and safety of budesonide/formoterol single inhaler therapy versus a higher dose of budesonide in moderate to severe Asthma. *Curr Medical Res Opin* 2004; 20: 1403–1418.

31. O'Byrne PM, Bisgaard H, Philippe P, *et al*. Budesonide/formoterol combination therapy as both maintenance and reliever medication in asthma. *Am J Resp Critical Care Med* 2005; 171: 129–136.

16

Compliance and concordance

The terms compliance, adherence and concordance are fundamentally different.[1]

- Compliance is defined as to the extent to which a patient follows the advice provided by a health professional. It implies that the patient *will* follow the instructions provided.
- Adherence focuses more on commitment to the medication regimen and involves limited negotiation between patient and professional.
- Concordance refers to a consultation process of prescribing and medicine-taking on the basis of a partnership between the prescriber and the patient. It is based on a notion of equality and respect for the patient and their autonomy and should consist of three components.[2]
    - Patients have enough knowledge to participate as partners.
    - Prescribing consultations involve patients as partners.
    - Patients are supported in taking medicines.

It is therefore possible to have a patient whom is non-compliant (or non-adherent) but not non-concordant. Only the consultation discussion between the patient and professional can be non-concordant.

The success of pharmacological treatment depends directly on the combined effectiveness of the treatment choice and compliance with the medication regimen – neither factor in isolation will produce successful disease management. If the patient is not given the most appropriate and effective medication, or if the patient is concordant but is given an inferior agent, treatment will not succeed.[3]

Poor compliance to medicine taking is not a new problem. It is recorded that around 200 BC, Hippocrates advised the physician, ". . . to be alert to the faults of the patients which make them lie about their taking of the medicines prescribed and when things go wrong, refuse to confess that they have not been taking their medicines."

Conservative estimates indicate that almost 50% of all prescription medications dispensed are not taken as prescribed.[4] Non-compliance or poor adherence to medical advice and treatments is a significant problem in patients with asthma and increases both mortality and morbidity in this population.[5,6] In one study of adults with mild-to-moderate asthma receiving treatment at steps 2 or 3 of the British Thoracic Society/ Scottish Intercollegiate Guidelines Network (BTS/SIGN) asthma management guideline the estimated adherence rate was 60% in adults aged 16–69 years, rising to 69% in older people. Adherence was only slightly better in patients with moderate-to-severe asthma (steps 4 or 5), at 66% and 73%, respectively, for the two age groups. Overall, 25% of patients had estimated adherence rates of 30% or less during the 5 years of the study.[7] Another study of patients with moderate or severe asthma found that 16% of users of inhaled beta-2 agonists reported over-use (more than eight puffs per day on days of use), and 64% of users of inhaled corticosteroids reported under-use (use on 4 days/week or fewer, or four puffs per day or fewer).[8]

Failure to follow an effective asthma management plan can have detrimental consequences. These include: unnecessary symptoms that could interfere with daily activities, acute exacerbations, airway re-modelling leading to 'fixed' airway disease,[9] deterioration in lung function, disability and death.

Improving concordance with medication can therefore have many benefits. Patients have the most to gain from improving their concordance with asthma treatment plans, leading to no or few symptoms and a dramatically improved quality of life. Health professionals will gain a sense of satisfaction in helping to reduce the costs of asthma to the individual and the National Health Service and preventing further complications.

Medication is only one aspect of concordance, particularly in the case of asthma management. Patients are asked to adhere to a number of management strategies:

- compliance with medication
- compliance with a written management plan
- attendance at follow-up appointments
- avoidance of allergy and trigger factors
- peak flow monitoring
- inhalational techniques
- recording of symptoms
- regular review.

Types of non-concordance

There are several types of non-concordance, as well as degrees or levels of compliance. Patient non-concordance with medication may be divided into primary non-concordance, where the patient for some reason fails to have the medicine dispensed, and secondary non-concordance, where the patient does not take the medication as prescribed. Identifying the type may help to establish the most appropriate form of intervention that will improve the patient's self-management and asthma control.

Primary non-concordance

This is when the patient does not get the prescription filled or fails to attend an appointment. Most studies have focused on secondary non-concordance. However, it is crucial to determine whether patients actually redeem their prescriptions from the pharmacy, because this is the first step in the complex phenomenon of concordance Studies on primary non-concordance indicate that primary non-compliance ranges from 6 to 44%.[10] However, these studies vary greatly in terms of assessment of primary non-concordance, participants and setting. A higher probability of primary non-concordance with medication rates are associated with individual characteristics such as younger age, financial strain, low self-related health and lack of trust in the healthcare system.[11]

Secondary non-concordance

As mentioned above, secondary non-concordance is where the patient does not take their medicine as intended. This category can be subdivided further.

Unintenional non-concordance

Unintentional non-concordance is where the patient may want to take a medicine but is prevented from doing so by barriers. For example, side-effects may be so immediate or severe that the drug has to be stopped. Simple issues can also lead to unintentional non-concordance, for example not being able to get the cap off a bottle or use an inhaler effectively. The patient may be unaware that they are not complying. For example, the patient doesn't realise that their inhaler technique is unlikely to deliver any of the drug to the lung, such as failure to remove the cap from the inhaler, to shake the inhaler or to breathe out when actuating a meter dose inhaler.

Asthma management plans, especially for severe disease, can be complex and patients may inadvertently be non-adherent because they do not fully understand the specifics of the regimen or the necessity for adherence. Patients frequently forget the instructions that they receive during consultations. In addition, inhalers do not usually have labels showing dosing instructions, and the labelled outer box is often discarded once opened. Patients may also interpret instructions such as "use medication twice a day" as "use medication twice a day when short of breath". Unintentional non-concordance can be corrected by improved communication between health professional and the patient.

Erratic non-concordance

Patients may have an erratic pattern of concordance, in which medication use alternates between fully concordant (usually when symptomatic) and under-use or total non-use (when asymptomatic). This is the most common form of non-concordance in patients with asthma.[10] Patients who are asymptomatic may have busy lifestyles, and changing schedules may interfere with compliance. The patient understands their regimen and often would like to comply appropriately but simply forgets to take their prescribed medication when well.

Patients with asthma may exhibit a different pattern of concordance for each of the medications they are prescribed. Many patients under-use the prescribed prophylactic anti-inflammatory (e.g. inhaled corticosteroids) medications while remaining appropriately adherent with other medications.[12] By relying solely on short-acting beta-2 agonists for symptomatic relief, the patient may delay seeking further care during exacerbations or may experience complications associated with excessive use of beta-2 agonists (see Chapter 10).

Strategies to improve erratic concordance involve simplifying the regimen (e.g. once-daily dosing), establishing a new routine through linking (e.g. keeping the inhaler next to the toothbrush) and use of cues and memory aids (e.g. tablet organisers).

Intentional non-concordance

Sometimes patients purposely discontinue or change the dose of their medications. This deliberate non-concordance is called intentional non-concordance, reflecting a reasoned choice, rather than necessarily a sensible one. Research has shown that these 'to-take-or-not-to-take' decisions are influenced by patient beliefs. Patients who are asymptomatic may decide they no longer need to take prescribed medication. This may be because they fear dependence or side-effects from treatment or the stigma or embarrassment associated with using an inhaler in public, or simply because they cannot afford the prescription charge for the drugs and devices. Fear of perceived short- or long-term side-effects of inhaled corticosteroids is a well-documented reason for patients reducing or discontinuing dosing.[12,13] For those patients the disadvantages of therapy outweigh the benefits.

Intentional non-concordance is where the move from compliance to concordance may lead to improved management for individual patients.[1] The prescriber may have to accept that compromise may be the best solution for the individual.

Factors affecting concordance with treatment

Many factors constantly influence the patient and their behaviour and choices in relation to managing their asthma (see Risk Factor Focus, page 244). The medical argument for concordance with medication competes with personal, social, cultural and lifestyle factors, which may change over time and asthma severity. Every patient will have different beliefs about their asthma, their daily routines, the goal of therapy and their capacity to adhere. These factors need to be taken into consideration when giving advice, prescribing or dispensing medication or providing education about asthma.[13,14]

Medication-related factors

Concordance with a drug regimen is reduced when the frequency of administration exceeds twice a day. There is, however, little difference between once- and twice-daily drug regimens and, in some cases, twice-daily dosing may preferable because forgetting a tablet has less therapeutic effect than forgetting a once-daily tablet.[10,15] Nevertheless, administration of asthma therapy only once a day has been shown to be preferable to most patients – 61% of patients expressed a preference for once-daily treatment compared with 12% who preferred twice daily dosing (27% expressed no preference).[16] While preference may not necessarily lead to improved concordance, it may reduce the burden of therapy and enhance the patient's quality of life.

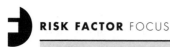

RISK FACTOR FOCUS

Factors contributing to poor adherence to asthma treatment

Patient-related factors

- Misunderstanding treatment and/or condition
- Forgetfulness
- Personal beliefs
- Denial or self-neglect
- Mood disorder (e.g. depression, anxiety, panic attacks)
- Substance abuse
- Embarrassment about their asthma
- Lack of social support
- Inability to afford prescription charges
- Unwillingness to pay prescription charges
- Language barriers

Treatment-related factors

- Fear or experience of adverse effects
- Complex regimen
- Frequent dosing
- Inconvenient dosing schedule
- Method of administration (patient unable to manage method or dislikes method)

Condition-related factors

- No or mild symptoms
- Severe symptoms

The more complex the treatment regimen, the easier it is for the patient to make a mistake and unintentionally not adhere. Drug regimens that involve multiple drugs with different routes of administration or different inhalers that require different inhalation techniques will reduce concordance with therapy. Polypharmacy is a well-recognised problem, particularly for many elderly patients. Therefore, when managing asthma, the general aim should be to keep the regimen as simple as possible.

Patients (or parents) who have concerns about using their medications may not comply appropriately. Patients and parents frequently have misconceptions about the function, adverse effects and long-term consequences of inhaled corticosteroids. For example, in one study over 40% of patients believed that inhaled corticosteroids opened up the airways to relieve bronchoconstriction, while fewer than a quarter of the patients realised that inhaled corticosteroids reduced airway inflammation. Of the patients interviewed, 46% indicated they were reluctant to use inhaled corticosteroids regularly but only 25% had discussed their fears and concerns about inhaled corticosteroids with a health professional.[17]

It is important that patients understand how their medication works, and particularly the difference between preventer and reliever medications. Patients should be shown how to use their medication devices and have their technique checked regularly, and should receive information about possible adverse effects.

Interventions to improve concordance

Identifying the presence and type of non-concordance will allow the health professional to develop an appropriate strategy to improve concordance. A commitment to partnership between the health professional and patient will foster communication and encourage the patient to take control of their self-management. The best approach when managing non-concordance is to work with the patient towards a relationship based on knowledge and understanding, in which the patient's individual beliefs and attitudes are discussed and addressed in an open, non-judgemental way. Focusing on the positive benefits of good concordance, rather than the negative consequences of poor concordance, and devising practical strategies to address the burden of treatment on the patient's life, will help to achieve a positive outcome (see Management Focus, below).

MANAGEMENT FOCUS

Strategies to improve compliance with medication[6,10,14,18,19]

- Develop open, communicative, non-judgemental relationships with patients
  - Use open-ended questions at the beginning of the consultation
  - Avoid questions that elicit a yes/no response or that are judgemental in tone
  - Show empathy and warmth; follow-up on the patient's verbal and body language clues
  - Ask questions that will elicit information about the patient's health beliefs, their attitude to their diagnosis and their willingness to make behavioural changes in order to manage their asthma better
  - Normalise non-compliance – remember about 50% of patients do not comply with prescribed medication regimens

Continued overleaf

Management Focus 16.1 (continued)

- Adopt a partnership approach to asthma management with your patient (concordance)
- Involve your patient in the planning process and tailor the final treatment plan to your patient's preferences, needs and capabilities
- Simplify treatment regimens where possible
- Ensure that your patient understands their asthma and treatment
- Ensure that your patient understands the benefits of complying with their medication: compliance will give them control, rather than asthma controlling them
- Explain likely adverse effects and discuss ways in which these can be minimised
- Always provide an opportunity for patients to express any concerns about the medication
- Present a written treatment plan, supplementing with verbal instructions
- Repeat instructions
- Use reminders:
  - individualised reminder charts
  - diaries
  - engage family members and carers to provide reminders
- If strategies or treatments have an unsatisfactory result, encourage the patient not to see this as a failure
- Collaborate with other healthcare professionals to improve patient outcomes
- Don't try to instruct patients in all aspects of asthma at one consultation – build their knowledge base over consecutive visits; present the most important information first, as this is best retained by the patient
- Emphasising disease severity will not necessarily improve adherence – helping a patient to realise how good they are likely to feel is more likely to be successful

References

1. Marinker M. From compliance to concordance: achieving shared goals in medicine taking. London: Royal Pharmaceutical Society; 1998.
2. Weiss M, Britten N. "What is concordance?" *Pharm J* 2003; 271: 493.
3. Anon. Are you taking the medicines? *Lancet* 1990; 335: 262–263.
4. Clepper I. Non-compliance, the invisible epidemic. *Drug Topics* 1992; 17: 44–65.
5. Juniper EF. The impact of patient compliance on effective asthma management. *Curr Opin Pulmon Med* 2003; 9 (Suppl 1): S8–S10.
6. O'Connor B. Optimising asthma control and concordance in adults. *Airways J* 2005; 3: 204–6.
7. Das Gupta R, Guest JF. Factors affecting UK primary care costs of managing patients with asthma over 5 years. *Pharmacoeconomics* 2003; 21: 357–369.

8. Diette GB, Wu AW, Skinner EA, *et al.* Treatment patterns among adult patients with asthma: factors associated with overuse of inhaled beta-agonists and under use of inhaled corticosteroids. *Arch Intern Med* 1999; 159: 2697–2704.

9. Redington AE, Howarth PH. Airway wall remodelling in asthma. (editorial). *Thorax* 1997; 52: 310–312.

10. World Health Organization. *Adherence to long term therapies: Evidence for action.* Geneva; WHO, 2003

11. Johnell K, Lindstrom M, Sundquist J, *et al.* Individual characteristics, area social participation, and primary non-concordance with medication: a multi-level analysis. *BMC Public Health* 2006; 6: 52.

12. Cochrane MC, Bala MV, Downs KE, *et al.* Inhaled corticosteroids for asthma therapy: patient compliance, devices and inhalation technique. *Chest* 2000; 117: 542–550.

13. Bosley CM, Fosbury JA, Cochrane GM. The psychological factors associated with poor compliance with treatment in asthma. *Eur Respir J* 1995; 8: 899–904.

14. Haynes RB, McDonald H, Garg AX, *et al.* Interventions for helping patients to follow prescriptions for medications. *The Cochrane Library*, issue 3. Chichester: John Wiley & Sons, 2001 (www.thecochranelibrary.com).

15. Weiner P, Weiner M, Azgad Y. Long term clinical comparison of single versus twice daily administration of inhaled budesonide in moderate asthma. *Thorax* 1995; 50: 1270–1273.

16. Venables TL, Addlestone MB, Smithers AJ, *et al.* A comparison of the efficacy and patient acceptability of once daily budesonide via Turbohaler and twice daily fluticasone propionate via disc inhaler at an equal daily dose of 400 micrograms in adult asthmatics. *Br J Clin Res* 1996; 7: 15–32.

17. Boulet LP. Perception of the role and potential side effects of inhaled corticosteroids among asthmatics patients. *Chest* 1998; 113: 587–592.

18. British Thoracic Society/Scottish Intercollegiate Guidelines Network. British Guideline on the Management of Asthma. *Thorax* 2003; 58 (Suppl I): S1–S94.

19. Schraa JC, Dirks JF. Improving patient recall and comprehension of the treatment regimen. *J Asthma* 1981; 19: 159–162.

17

Role of the pharmacist in the management of asthma

With good asthma care, patients experience fewer symptoms and improved quality of life, as well as fewer hospital admissions and exacerbations. The responsibility for good asthma care is a team effort, both in primary and secondary care. All members of the healthcare team should work in collaboration to achieve the goals of asthma management and improve patient outcomes (see Management Focus, Chapter 3, page 32).

Many factors have been found to be associated with poor outcomes in asthma, including non-concordance (see Chapter 16), improper inhaler technique (see Chapter 7), ignorance of prescribing guidelines (see Chapters 3 and 4), poor follow-up, inadequate use of corticosteroids (see Chapters 3 and 16) and poverty. Pharmacists have the training to positively influence many of these factors and drive forwards improvements in asthma patient care.[1,2]

Aims of pharmacological management

The aims of pharmacological management of asthma are the control of symptoms, including nocturnal symptoms and exercise-induced asthma, prevention of exacerbations and the achievement of best possible pulmonary function, with minimal side-effects. The management of medicines is a specific role for pharmacists and they can help to achieve the aims of pharmacological management.

Role of the pharmacist

The delivery of care to an asthmatic patient is a complex process. Whether they work in community pharmacies, hospitals, or general practice clinics, pharmacists are in a pivotal position to contribute to the overall management of asthma. The pharmacist can contribute to patient care by identifying poorly controlled asthma, assessing inhaler technique, advising about smoking cessation if necessary and medicine management (including advice on over-the-counter medicines, minimising adverse effects and drug interactions and monitoring patient concordance). Pharmacists can also be a valuable source of important information for other members of the healthcare team.

The pharmacist, especially the community pharmacist, is an easily accessible source of advice for the patient and they are in a unique 'frontline' position to assess and monitor a patient's medication. The pharmacist is likely to see patients on long-term treatment plans more regularly than their general practitioner (GP) or practice nurse. Pharmacists can use these meetings as an opportunity to provide pharmaceutical care to the patient with asthma. Any patient the pharmacist is concerned about can be referred back to their GP or asthma specialist (see Management Focus, below).

The general medical service contract

Asthma is an important part of the clinical domain in the quality and outcomes framework of the new general medical service (GMS)

MANAGEMENT FOCUS 17.1

Patients who should be referred back to their doctor or asthma specialist

---

- Medicines not helping as they usually do
- Frequent or worsening symptoms
- Symptoms interfering with daily activities
- Frequent or worsening nocturnal symptoms
- Early morning wakening because of breathlessness or chest tightness
- Patients experiencing adverse effects of medication
- Consistently poor inhaler technique, requiring a more appropriate device
- Excessive use of short-acting beta-2 agonists prescribed on an as-needed basis (more than two canisters each month)
- Patients not filling prescriptions for inhaled corticosteroids or not using them regularly
- Patients frequently requesting emergency supplies of medications
- Prolonged winter cough that does not settle after antibiotic therapy
- Co-existent persistent rhinitis with respiratory symptoms
- Patient appears insecure, frustrated or is displaying fearful behaviour about their illness and/or treatment
- Possible undiagnosed symptoms in customers who regularly buy non-prescription medicines (e.g. a 'wheezy' patient requesting medicines containing theophylline)
- Prescription for medicines that may interact with concurrent medication

contract, ranking fourth in terms of points available (72) behind coronary heart disease, hypertension and diabetes (see the Appendix). A further 42 points are available for medicines management in the organisational domain of the contract. The new contract provides opportunities for pharmacists to work with GPs and practice managers to maximise the number of quality indicators achieved and to provide directly services not being provided by a practice. Examples of areas where pharmacists could be involved include:

- medication review
- establishing and maintaining disease registers
- review and advice on repeat-prescription systems and practice protocols
- adherence to the British Thoracic Society/Scottish Intercollegiate Guidelines Network (BTS/SIGN) asthma management guideline
- provision of smoking-cessation services
- support of influenza vaccination campaign
- provision of minor ailment schemes to help improve access to GPs
- supplementary prescribing services.

In 2005 a new community pharmacy contract was implemented. It is designed to help drive pharmacy care to new horizons and fully integrate it into the National Health Service. The contract allows pharmacists to move beyond traditional dispensing services to service developments such as those highlighted above (see Management Focus, page 250). The new scheme could benefit many people with asthma, who will be able to get a prescription from their GP lasting a year, and take it to their pharmacy as and when they need more medication. This provides a regular platform for conducting a medication review and providing advice on their asthma management plan.

Studies on pharmacist-based care

Numerous studies have shown the benefits of pharmacists becoming more involved in the care of patients with asthma, although few of these studies were based in the UK. A Danish study of community pharmacists working with physicians using a therapeutic outcomes management protocol showed beneficial effects on asthma symptoms, global and asthma-related quality of life, days of sickness, knowledge and inhaler technique, but not in peak flow rates.[3,4] One small Finnish community pharmacy study had an impact on a few outcome measures,[5] while a small Maltese study showed that a community-pharmacy-based asthma

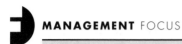

Ways in which pharmacists can become more involved in the care of patients with asthma

Simple interventions

- Briefly question patients on asthma symptoms and control
- Count repeat prescription requests to check whether patients are over-using their short-acting beta-2 agonists or under-using their inhaled corticosteroids
- Check inhaler technique
- Help patients to use peak flow meters appropriately
- Health promotion advice (e.g. smoking cessation)
- Lifestyle advice such as coping with coughs, colds or hay fever
- Encourage patients who want to purchase over-the counter medications to seek medical care if appropriate
- Help patients who are discharged from hospital to understand their asthma management plan and reinforce any changes
- Provide information about asthma medications

Detailed interventions

- Set up and run a medicine management clinic
- Become a supplementary prescriber in order to work with the general practitioner/hospital consultant to monitor asthma patients and step therapy up and down as appropriate
- Set up and run smoking cessation clinics for asthma patients
- Provide patients with self-action plans to manage their asthma
- Help general practices to meet the asthma quality targets in the new general medical services contract

education and monitoring program impacted on quality of life, pulmonary function, inhaler technique and the number of hospitalisations.[6] A study in New Zealand determined the impact of a community-pharmacy-based pharmaceutical care service to asthma patients. The service involved the creation of a patient record, identification of medication-related problems and development strategies to resolve these problems and monitor outcomes. The study showed that this service led to improvements in asthma management and quality of life for the majority of patients.[7] An American study reported less favourable results for pharmacists. It showed that pharmaceutical care provided by community pharmacists to patients with asthma (or chronic obstructive pulmonary disease) resulted in only slight improvements in lung function (measured by peak flow meters).[8] Furthermore; it resulted in an increase in the number of GP visits with breathing-related problems. However, the inclusion of patients with chronic obstructive pulmonary disease may have skewed the results.

A study in the UK investigated whether a community pharmacist with basic asthma training could improve asthma control with a simple programme of self-management advice.[9] Participants randomised to the intervention group (n = 12) received a review of their inhaler technique and personal education from the pharmacist, addressing topics such as basic asthma pathophysiology, recognition and avoidance of triggers, inhaler technique, self-management skills, including monitoring of peak flow or symptoms, action in response to worsening symptoms, how to access emergency care appropriately, and smoking cessation if relevant. Individual sessions lasted 45–60 minutes. The pharmacist telephoned the patients in the intervention group weekly, encouraging them to return to the pharmacy with any problems. The control group (n = 12) had no input from the pharmacist. After the 3-month study period, all but one participant in the intervention group reported an improvement in symptoms and the remaining participant's score was unchanged. Scores for participants in the control group worsened slightly overall. The study suggests that a community pharmacist with basic training in asthma care can deliver a simple educational programme, resulting in improvements in asthma control.

The benefits of pharmacist interventions in asthma were also shown in a pilot scheme by community pharmacists in the UK.[10] Pharmacists identified 'disuse and abuse of preventer inhalers' and 'regular use of reliever inhalers' in 58 out of the 103 patients involved. A total of 122 interventions were made and the patients' GPs were contacted where necessary.

Other studies have also shown that patients report an increased level of satisfaction with a service that includes a pharmacist, and that increased patient education, coupled with a comprehensive asthma health management programme, improve the process of care and the outcomes of treatment.[11–16]

Control of symptoms

Identification of poor control

The fact that so many asthma patients remain symptomatic suggests widespread under-assessment and, in some cases, under-treatment.

Symptomatic patients must be identified and referred to their medical practice for an assessment of their asthma, to ensure that they are being treated according to the correct step of the BTS/SIGN asthma management guideline.

Patients with asthma typically present repeatedly with respiratory symptoms – a recurring pattern of presentation that should alert the pharmacist. Community pharmacists should be prepared to question patients who present with regular prescriptions for cough medicines or antibiotics and patients who frequently purchase non-prescription medicines for respiratory conditions. Patients who request emergency supplies of respiratory medicines should also be questioned, and referred to their medical practice if necessary. Most community pharmacists have the facility to monitor repeat prescriptions and should be able to identify patients who are using more than two canisters of short-acting beta-2 agonists a month, which is indicative of poor control. It may also be possible to identify patients who are not filling their prescriptions for inhaled corticosteroids at regular intervals.

It is not possible to provide a standard assessment approach for pharmacists to manage people with asthma that would be appropriate for every situation. However, pharmacists may find it useful to adapt the checklists outlined in this chapter to suit their particular requirements.

Checklist for identification of poor asthma control

- Is the patient requesting frequent emergency supplies of respiratory medicines?
- Is the patient using more than two canisters of short acting beta-2 agonists each month? *See Chapter 16, page 24.*
- Has the patient had difficulty sleeping because of their asthma symptoms (including cough)? *See Monitoring Focus, Chapter 6, page 96.*
- Has the patient had their usual asthma symptoms during the day (cough, wheeze, chest tightness or breathlessness)? *See Monitoring Focus, Chapter 6, page 96.*
- Has their asthma interfered with their usual activities (e.g. housework, work, school etc)? *See Monitoring Focus, Chapter 6, page 96.*
- Does the patient notice that their symptoms are worse when at work? *See Diagnostic Focus, Chapter 2, page 15.*
- Does the patient find that their medicines are not helping as much as usual? *See Diagnostic Focus, Chapter 2, page 27, Diagnostic Focus,*

Chapter 4, pages 65–66, Risk Factors Focus, Chapter 2, page 12 and Management Focuses, Chapter 8, pages 141–143.

Education

Pharmacists can help patients understand that, with appropriate therapy, it is usually possible to lead a normal, productive and physically active life. Educating the patient may help to allay their fears and improve concordance with their medication. Every consultation with a patient with asthma is an opportunity to review, reinforce and extend both knowledge and skills. It is important to realise that education is an ongoing process, not a single event.

Checklist for providing patient education

- Are there any potential barriers that may influence the outcome of providing information to the patient? *See Management Focus, Chapter 8, page 134.*
- Does the patient know the role of each of their medicines? *See Table 10.2 (page 156–158), Table 10.3 (page 159), Table 10.4 (page 161–162), Table 12.2 (page 196–198), Management Focus, Chapter 12, page 180, Monitoring Focus, Chapter 13, page 204, Table 13.1 (page 212–213) and Management Focus, Chapter 14, page 217, Table 14.1 (page 221).*
- Does the patient know that preventative medication should be taken on a regular basis, even when they are free of symptoms? *See Chapter 12, page 187.*
- Does the patient know that short-acting beta-2 agonists should be used when required for shortness of breath? *See Chapter 6, page 109.*
- Does the patient know how to take their medicine, how much to take and how often?
- Does the patient know how to evaluate response to therapy? *See Monitoring Focuses, Chapter 6, pages 96 and 98.*
- Does the patient know when to seek medical care and what to do if the desired effect is not achieved or side-effects are encountered? *See Management Focuses, Chapter 8, pages 141–143.*
- Does the patient understand their asthma action plan? *See Chapter 8, page 140.*
- Does the patient use the proper technique for inhaling their medications? *See Chapter 7.*
- Does the patient use the proper technique for their peak flow meter? *See Monitoring Focus, Chapter 6, page 98.*

Promoting patient concordance with medication

Now that pharmacists can become supplementary prescribers, they can take full responsibility for concordance, since the major thrust of the concept is achieved within the consultation during which the decision to prescribe is made.

Pharmacists in more traditional roles are also important in promoting patient concordance with medication – concordance is not possible if the patient is not well-informed. Pharmacists have the expertise to educate patients about their medications and disease status. They are usually the first port of call for patients with a new prescription. Pharmacists should take this opportunity to ensure that the patient understands why the particular medicine has been prescribed and that they are satisfied with the decision. This includes an awareness of adverse effects and the potential benefits of treatment. Counselling when handing over medicines should not merely include advice about the when and how of compliance, but should also actively seek feedback from the patient on their medication beliefs, encouraging a concordant relationship. It is important to realise that some patients may not want to be involved in concordance and would rather be told what to take.

Prescribers must have the basic knowledge required to inform their patients about their medications. Concordance must continue throughout the course of the disease, and medication review is essential to ensure that the patient is still satisfied with treatment and that they do not require any alterations. This includes an understanding of the attainment of outcomes. The role of the pharmacist in medication review has been reflected positively in the new pharmacy contract of 2005.

Concordance is as important with over-the-counter medicines as for prescription-only medicines. Patients who seek advice should receive as much information as they need or want to ensure safe and effective self-treatment. For concordance to be meaningful, all health professionals caring for a particular patient must understand why certain treatment decisions have been made. Pharmacists are in an excellent position to share details of the medication history and reasons for changes in medications with other health professionals across the primary/secondary care interface.

Checklist for promoting concordance with medication

- Are there any potential barriers that may influence the outcome of providing information to the patient with asthma? *See Management Focus, Chapter 8, page 134.*

- Are there any factors that may contribute to poor compliance with asthma medications? *See Risk Factors Focus, Chapter 16, page 244.*
- Is the patient using more than two canisters of short-acting beta-2 agonists per month? *See Chapter 16, page 242.*
- Does the patient know how to take their medication, how much to take and how often?
- Is the patient getting the correct inhaler or generic prescription? (Although generic prescribing is actively encouraged in the UK, there is the risk that patients will be provided with an unfamiliar device that they have not been trained to use. This will risk poor technique with potential for inadequate dosing and loss of asthma control.)[17]
- Does the patient understand the information given to them by their doctor or nurse?
- Is the patient aware of the long-term consequences of not taking their preventer medication? *See Figure 2.2, page 8 and Chapter 2, page 11.*
- Are there any strategies that could be employed to improve the patient's concordance? *See Management Focus, Chapter 16, page 245.*

Maximising lung function

An important aim of asthma management is to achieve and maintain the best possible lung function. Pharmacists can help to accomplish this aim by encouraging the prescribing of appropriate medication (in particular inhaled corticosteroids), by promoting patient concordance with their medication and asthma action plan, and by promoting a healthy lifestyle that includes exercise, appropriate diet and avoidance of tobacco smoke.

Checklist to help maximise lung function

- Is the patient on the step of the BTS/SIGN asthma management guideline that is appropriate to their disease severity? *See Figures 3.1, 3.2 and 3.3, pages 34–36.*
- Has the patient's medication been reviewed recently?
- Does the patient need an increase in treatment (step up) to improve asthma control? *See Figures 3.1, 3.2 and 3.3, pages 34–36.*
- Has smoking-cessation advice been offered (where applicable)? *See Figure 5.1, Chapter 5, page 85.*
- Does the patient know which trigger factors to avoid and how to avoid them? *See Risk Factors Focus, Chapter 2, page 12 and Management Focus, Chapter 5, page 83.*

- Does the patient know that preventer medication should be taken on a regular basis even when they are free of symptoms? *See Chapter 12, page 187.*
- Is the patient aware of the long-term consequences of not taking their preventer medication? *See Figure 2.2, page 8.*
- Does the patient have an optimal inspiratory flow volume for their prescribed inhaler? *See Inhalation Delivery Focus, Chapter 7, page 117.*
- Would the patient with asthma benefit from using a spacer device with their inhaler? *See Inhalation Delivery Focus, Chapter 7, page 118.*

Prevention of exacerbations

Mortality and morbidity from asthma exacerbations can be reduced by educating the patient about their condition and treatments, encouraging patient self-management and improving the organisation of patient care in both primary and secondary care. Early detection of exacerbations, through improved communications between the patient and health professionals, will also hopefully reduce decline in lung function and hospitalisation rates.

Checklist to help prevent exacerbations of asthma

- Is the patient at high risk of developing near-fatal or fatal asthma? *See Risk Factors Focus, Chapter 4, page 59.*
- Does the patient have signs and symptoms that could indicate an exacerbation? *See Chapter 4, page 63, Diagnostic Focus, Chapter 4, page 65.*
- Can the patient correctly interpret the warning symptoms of an acute exacerbation at home and adjust treatments accordingly? *See Diagnostic Focus, Chapter 4, page 65 and Management Focuses, Chapter 8, pages 141–143.*
- Does the patient know when to seek medical care and what to do when the desired effect is not achieved? *See Management Focus, Chapter 8, page 141.*
- Does the patient have an effective asthma action plan? *See Management Focuses, Chapter 8, pages 141–143.*
- Does the patient understand their asthma action plan? *See Chapter 8, page 140.*
- Does the patient use the proper technique for inhaling their medications? *See Chapter 7.*
- Does the patient know which medicines are used to prevent and/or decrease the frequency of asthma symptoms?

- Does the patient know that their preventer medication should be taken on a regular basis even when they are free of symptoms? *See Chapter 12, page 187.*
- Does the patient know which trigger factors to avoid and how to avoid them? *See Risk Factors Focus, Chapter 2, page 12 and Management Focus, Chapter 5, page 83.*
- Has smoking-cessation advice been offered (where applicable)? *See Figure 5.1, Chapter 5, page 85.*
- Is the patient with an acute exacerbation of asthma being treated according to the BTS/SIGN asthma management guideline? *See Figures 4.2 and 4.3, pages 67 and 74.*
- Has the patient received a pneumococcal vaccine? *See Chapter 3, page 52.*
- Has the patient received their annual influenza vaccination? *See Chapter 3, page 53.*

Minimising adverse effects

The aims of pharmacological management of asthma are the control of symptoms, prevention of exacerbations and the achievement of best possible pulmonary function, with *minimal adverse effects*. The pharmacist can help to minimise adverse effects by ensuring effective medication management, screening for drug interactions and by being aware of problems associated with medicines.

Medication management involves the pharmacist working with GPs and patients to help patients get the most from their medicines in order to maintain or improve their quality and duration of life. This is achieved through ensuring that patients do not suffer from illness or adverse effects because of inappropriate or inadequate therapy; ensuring that medication is optimised early in the treatment programme, supporting patients in using medicines and empowering them to manage their own care.

Checklist for effective medicines management

- Is the patient on the step of the asthma guidelines appropriate to their disease severity? *See Figures 3.1, 3.2 and 3.3, pages 34–36.*
- Is the patient on the correct dose of inhaled corticosteroid for their disease severity? *See Management Focus, Chapter 3, Figures 3.1, 3.2 and 3.3, pages 34–36 and Figure 12.3, page 186.*
- Would the patient benefit from using a spacer device with their inhaler? *See Inhalation Delivery Focus, Chapter 7, page 118.*

- Is the patient's asthma stable, such that their treatments could be decreased (step down)? *See Figures 3.1, 3.2 and 3.3, pages 34–36.*
- Does the patient require a steroid warning card (prolonged or frequent courses of oral corticosteroids or taking more than 1 mg/day inhaled beclometasone or equivalent)? *Chapter 12, page 193.*
- Does the patient have any noticeable adverse effects from their medications? *See Adverse Effects Focus, Chapter 3, page 44, Adverse Effects Focus, Chapter 10, page 166, Adverse Effects Focus, Chapter 11, page 174, Adverse Effect Focus, Chapter 12, page 189, Monitoring Focuses, Chapter 13, pages 204 and 210 and Adverse Effects Focus, Chapter 14, page 222.*
- Is any patient taking a methylxanthine preparation aware of:
  - the possible drug interactions with methylxanthines? *See Risk Factors Focus, Chapter 13, page 211*
  - the factors that affect plasma theophylline levels? *See Risk Factors Focus, Chapter 13, page 206 and Management Focus, Chapter 13, page 207*
  - the need for careful monitoring of blood levels? *See Monitoring Focus, Chapter 13, page 204 and Management Focus, Chapter 13, page 205.*
- Does the patient have any factors that may affect methylxanthine metabolism? *See Risk Factors Focus, Chapter 13, page 206 and Management Focus, Chapter 13, page 207.*
- Is the prescribing of nebuliser medication appropriate for the patient? *See Inhalation Delivery Focus Chapter 7, page 126.*
- Is any patient using a nebuliser aware that:
  - the nebuliser compressor should be serviced regularly (at least once a year)?
  - a mouthpiece is the preferred method for delivery of nebulised drugs to the lungs? *See Chapter 7, page 129*
  - the nebuliser delivers a similar percentage of drug to the lungs as a metered-dose inhaler combined with a spacer device? *See Chapter 7, page 127.*
- Are there any clinical significant drug interactions in the patient's medication regimen? *See Chapter 10, page 165, Chapter 12, page 195, Chapter 13, page 209, Chapter 14, page 223 and Risk Factors Focus, Chapter 13, page 211.*

Checklist for use of pharmacy medicines

- Does the patient have known sensitivity to aspirin? *See Chapter 2, page 16 and Adverse Effects Focus, Chapter 17, page 261.*
- Is the patient taking any concurrent non-prescription medications that may potentially cause problems? *See Adverse Effects Focus, Chapter 17, page 261.*

ADVERSE EFFECTS FOCUS

Potential problems with over-the-counter medicines in asthma

Analgesics

- With an increase in the number of non-steroidal anti-inflammatory drugs (NSAIDs) available without a prescription, more people use such medications, increasing the potential for adverse reactions in people who are sensitive to aspirin. People with known sensitivity to aspirin need to be warned of the possibility of adverse reactions from commonly available pain relievers and low-dose aspirin. Adverse effects can occur from topical and oral products. Patients with known sensitivity should avoid any preparation containing aspirin. It is difficult to produce recommendations for a cohort of individuals with asthma who have never been exposed to NSAIDs.
- The concurrent use of oral corticosteroids and NSAIDs requires the patient to be monitored carefully because of the increased risk of gastrointestinal bleeding and ulceration.

Could and cough remedies

- Many contain NSAIDs – see above.
- Some contain theophylline (e.g. Do-Do Chesteze) – patients taking theophylline or aminophylline should not take other medications that contain theophylline unless the total dose of theophylline can be adjusted appropriately.

Antacids

The absorption of prednisolone can be reduced by large doses of aluminium or magnesium hydroxide antacids. Concurrent use should be monitored to ensure continued therapeutic response.

Histamine H2 antagonists

Cimetidine raises theophylline serum levels and toxicity may develop if the theophylline dose is not reduced. Initial reductions of 30–50% have been suggested. Other H2 antagonists (e.g. ranitidine) occasionally interact in a similar way.

Continued

Adverse Effects Focus (continued)

Proton pump inhibitors

Omeprazole when taken concurrently with enteric-coated prednisolone may cause the enteric coating to dissolve prematurely in the stomach, which may increase the risk of adverse gastrointestinal effects.

Caffeine

Caffeine can raise serum theophylline levels and may lead to adverse effects in a minority of individuals. Patients taking theophylline do not normally need to avoid caffeine (in over-the-counter medicines, coffee, tea, cola, etc.), but caffeine may occasionally be responsible for otherwise unexplained adverse effects.

Nicotine replacement therapy (NRT)

Tobacco smokers (and non-smokers heavily exposed to smoke) may need more theophylline than non-smokers to achieve the same therapeutic benefits because the theophylline is cleared from the body more quickly. However, this does NOT occur in those who chew NRT gum or use other NRT products.

References

1. Wilcock M, Mackenzie IF, White M,, et al.. How can the community pharmacist help the asthma patient? *Pharm J* 1999; 262; 815–816.
2. Wilcock M. How the community pharmacist can help. *Asthma J* 1997; 2: 71–72.
3. Herborg H, Soendergaard B, Froekjaer B, *et al.* Improving drug therapy for patients with asthma – part 1: patient outcomes. *J Am Pharm Assoc* 2001; 41: 539–550.
4. Herborg H, Soendergaard B, Froekjaer B, *et al.* Improving drug therapy for patients with asthma – part 2: use of antiasthma medications. *J Am Pharm Assoc* 2001; 41: 551–559.
5. Narhi U, Airaksinen M, Tanskanen P, *et al.* Therapeutic outcomes monitoring by community pharmacists for improving clinical outcomes in asthma. *J Clin Pharm Ther* 2000; 288: 1594–1602.
6. Cordina M, McElnay JC, Hughes CM. Assessment of a community pharmacy based programme for patients with asthma. *Pharmacotherapy* 2001; 21: 1196–1203.
7. Shaw JP, Emmerton L, Kheir NA, *et al.* Pharmaceutical care of asthma patients in a New Zealand community pharmacy setting. *Pharm J* 2000; 265: R24.
8. Weinberger M, Murray MD, Marrero DG, *et al.* Effectiveness of pharmacist care for patients with reactive airways disease: a randomised controlled trial. *JAMA* 2002; 288: 1594–1602.
9. Barbanel D, Eldridge S, Griffiths C. Can a self-management programme

delivered by a community pharmacist improve asthma control? A randomised trial. *Thorax* 2003; 58: 851–854.

10. National Association of Primary Care and National Pharmaceutical Association. Working with pharmacists to improve health. *Pharm J* 1999; 263: 721–722.

11. Knoell DL, Pierson JF, Marsh CB, *et al.* Measurement of outcomes in adults receiving pharmaceutical care in a comprehensive outpatient clinic. *Pharmacotherapy* 1998; 18: 1365–1374.

12. National education and prevention programme. The role of the pharmacist in improving asthma care. *Am Pharm* 1995; 35: 24–29.

13. Buchner DA, Butt L, De Stefano A, *et al.* Effects of an asthma management program on the asthmatic member: patient centred results of a two-year study in a managed care organisation. *Am J Managed Care* 1998; 4: 1288–1297.

14. Cote J, Cartier A, Robichaud P, *et al.* Influence on asthma morbidity of asthma education programs based on self-management plans following treatment optimization. *Am J Resp Crit Care Med* 1997; 155: 1509–1514.

15. Kradjan WA, Schula R, Christensen DB, *et al.* Patients' perceived benefit from and satisfaction with asthma-related pharmacy services. *Am J Pharm Assoc* 1999; 39: 658–666.

16. Cairns C, Eveleigh M. Community pharmacists' contribution to managing patients with asthma. *Asthma J* 2000; 5: 80–83.

17. Buchanan A, Pinnock H, Barnes J, *et al.* Generic prescribing of breath actuated and dry powder inhalers in the UK. *Prim Care Respir J* 2002; 11: 95.

Appendix

Asthma indicators in the general medical service contract

Asthma indicators		Points	Maximum threshold* (%)
Records			
ASTHMA 1	Production of a register of patients with asthma[†]	7	
Initial management			
ASTHMA 2	Diagnosis confirmed by spirometry or peak flow measurement (patients aged ≥8, diagnosed from 1 April 2003)	15	70
Ongoing management			
ASTHMA 3	Record of smoking status (patients aged 14–19)**	6	70
ASTHMA 4	Record of smoking status (patients aged ≥20)**	6	70
ASTHMA 5	Smoking cessation advice**	6	70
ASTHMA 6	Asthma review**	20	70
ASTHMA 7	Influenza vaccination in proceeding 1 September–31 March (patients aged ≥16)	12	70

[†]excluding patients who have been prescribed no asthma-related drugs in previous 12 months.
*minimum threshold: 25%.
**measured in previous 15 months.

Continued

Repeat prescribing indicators		*Points*	*Standard (%)*
Records and information			
RECORDS 9	For repeat medicines, an indication for the drug can be identified in the records (for drugs added to repeat prescription with effect from 1 April 2004)	4	80*
Medicines management			
MED 5	Medication review recorded in notes in previous 15 months for all patients being prescribed four or more repeat medicines	7	80
MED 9	Medication review recorded in notes in previous 15 months for all patients taking prescribed repeat medicines	8	80

*minimum standard.

Glossary

Agonist: a drug that binds to and activates receptors, producing a response.

Airway remodelling: the chronic inflammation of asthma can lead to irreversible airway remodelling, which is characterised by increased mucus, epithelial damage, basement membrane fibrosis, and fibroblast and smooth muscle cell hypertrophy and hyperplasia.

Allergen: a foreign substance that induces an allergy or hypersensitivity reaction in some individuals.

Alveoli: the blind-ending air sacs at the end of the respiratory tree that act as the primary gas exchange units of the lung.

Anaphylaxis: a severe allergic reaction to a foreign substance.

Antagonist: a drug that binds to receptors without activating them, and prevents access of agonists. The antagonism may be competitive or irreversible.

Antigen: an agent, usually a foreign protein, that causes a specific immune response.

Apnoea: absence of breathing.

Asphyxia: suffocation; a life-threatening condition in which oxygen cannot reach the tissues because of obstruction or damage to any part of the respiratory system.

Atopic: used to describe someone who has generated specific IgE against one or more allergens, as defined by a positive skin-prick test or *in vitro* test for specific IgE (e.g. RAST test).

Atopic disease: a disease related to a specific IgE response to allergens. The atopic diseases include atopic (extrinsic) asthma, atopic dermatitis (eczema) and allergic rhinitis.

Atopy: the tendency (inherited or constitutional) to develop hypersensitivity reactions such as asthma, eczema and hay fever.

Bronchial hyperresponsiveness: increased sensitivity of the airways to a variety of physical, chemical and pharmacological stimuli.

Bronchiectasis: an irreversible condition marked by chronic abnormal dilation of bronchi and destruction of bronchial walls.

Bronchiole: a smaller airway without cartilage.

Bronchoconstriction: narrowing of the airways that causes obstruction of airflow (sometimes termed airflow limitation).

Bronchodilation: widening of the smaller airways, allowing more air to flow in and out of the lungs.

Chemokines: a family of chemotactic cytokines that have the ability to attract and activate white blood cells.

Chemotaxis: the movement of cells in a particular direction in response to a chemical stimulus.

Concordance: a way to define the process of successful prescribing and medicine taking, based on a partnership between the patient and the healthcare professional.

Cyclic AMP: a second messenger that activates protein kinase A and is linked to the adenylate cyclase signal transduction pathway.

Cystic fibrosis: a hereditary disease affecting cells of the exocrine glands (including mucus-secreting glands, sweat glands and others).

Cytokines: proteins that modulate cellular immunity and are released mainly by activated lymphocytes and macrophages in response to a stimulus. Examples of cytokines are interleukins (produced by leukocytes), lymphokines (produced by lymphocytes), interferons and tumour necrosis factors.

Cytochrome P450 (CYP) isoenzymes: a family of isoenzymes in the liver that metabolise and detoxify various compounds, including many drugs.

Dyspnoea: difficulty breathing or a feeling of uncomfortable breathing.

Eosinophil: a type of white blood cell distinguished by the coarse granules in the cytoplasm that stain orange–red with Romanowsky stains. Eosinophils accumulate at sites of inflammation and release inflammatory mediators.

Eosinophilia: an increase in the number of eosinophils in the blood.

Extracorporeal membrane oxygenation (ECMO):   a technique used as a rescue treatment for potentially fatal respiratory failure. It involves modified prolonged cardiopulmonary bypass to support gas exchange, which allows the lungs to rest and recover.

Extrinsic (atopic) asthma   people whose symptoms are brought on by one or more external factors such as pollen or dust (allergens) are said to have allergic or extrinsic asthma. This is particularly common in children who develop asthma.

Histamine: an inflammatory mediator. It is one of the substances responsible for the swelling and redness associated with inflammation. Other effects include narrowing of the airways and itching.

Hypercapnia: an abnormally high concentration of carbon dioxide in the blood.

Hyperplasia: the increased production and growth of normal cells in a tissue or organ. The affected part becomes larger but retains its normal form.

Hypertrophy: increase in the size of a tissue or organ brought about by the enlargement of its cells rather than by cell multiplication.

Hyperventilation syndrome: breathing at an abnormally rapid rate at rest. This reduces the arterial carbon dioxide concentration, leading to dizziness, paraesthesiae in the lips and limbs, tetanic cramps in the hands and tightness across the chest.

Hypocapnia: an abnormally low concentration of carbon dioxide in the blood.

Hypoxaemia: reduced concentration of oxygen in arterial blood, recognised clinically by the presence of central and peripheral cyanosis.

Immunoglobulin E antibodies: protein–sugar complexes that are produced by the body in response to the presence of an antigen and combine with the foreign substance to make it harmless.

Immunotherapy: the prevention or treatment of disease using agents that may modify the immune response.

Interleukins: a group of molecules (cytokines) produced by white blood cells. They are involved in signalling between cells of the immune system.

Intrinsic asthma: people whose symptoms do not seem to be brought on by anything external are said to have non-allergic or intrinsic asthma. It is more common in people who develop asthma for the first time in adulthood. Symptoms are likely to be triggered by, for example, exercise, emotion or some drugs such as aspirin.

Leukotrienes: inflammatory mediators produced by white blood cells and macrophages that mediate the inflammation associated with allergic and asthmatic reactions.

Lymphocytes: another name for white blood cells. They form part of the body's immune system and play an important role in defending the body against invading organisms. There are two types: B lymphocytes and T lymphocytes (described below).

Macrophages: cells that filter and remove foreign particles from the body, secrete cytokines and activate lymphocytes.

Mast cells: cells that release histamine and other chemicals involved in inflammation.

Monoclonal antibodies: antibodies produced artificially from a cell clone, that recognise the same antigenic epitope.

Neutrophils: white blood cells that defend the body against invading organisms, such as bacteria and viruses. Neutrophils move to the site of infection or inflammation, where they ingest and destroy the invading organism.

Paradoxical breathing: breathing movements that are the reverse of normal: the chest wall moves in on inspiration and out on expiration. Patients with chronic airways obstruction show indrawing of the lower ribs during inspiration because of the distorted action of a depressed and flattened diaphragm.

Paradoxical bronchospasm: the apparently contradictory narrowing of the airways following the inhalation of a drug that is intended to relax the airways (e.g. beta-2 agonists).

Platelet-activating factor (PAF):   a substance produced in response to specific stimuli by activated platelets, neutrophils and basophils in the blood. PAF stimulates platelets to clump together and form blood clots, and also induces bronchoconstriction.

Pneumothorax: presence of air in the pleural cavity.

Prostaglandins: naturally occurring chemicals in the body that act as hormones. Prostaglandins are found in many different tissues and have a wide range of effects in the body, including causing pain and inflammation in damaged tissues and the development of fever.

Rhinosinusitis: inflammation of the lining of the nose and paranasal sinuses.

Sarcoidosis: a multisystem granulomatous disorder.

Skin-prick tests: test to identify specific IgEs, in which the skin is scratched lightly with a needle through a drop of allergen extract. A positive reaction is characterised by wheal and flare, the size of the wheal being taken as a measure of the size of the response.

Sympathomimetics: drugs that partially or completely mimic the actions of noradrenaline (norepinephrine) and adrenaline (epinephrine).

Tachypnoea: shallow breathing at increased respiratory rate.

T lymphocytes: white blood cells found in blood and the lymphatic system that are involved in cell-mediated immunity. Following activation by the presence of an invading organism, the T lymphocytes migrate to the site of the antigen, where they either destroy it or activate other immune cells to do so.

Tumour necrosis factor (TNF):   a cytokine that acts as a messenger between cells of the immune system. It is produced by white blood cells in response to infection or the presence of cancer cells, and activates white blood cells to seek and destroy foreign substances. TNF also causes inflammation in asthma and rheumatoid arthritis.

Tumour necrosis factor-alpha (TNF-alpha):   a member of the TNF family of cytokine proteins.

Useful resources

Websites

Asthma UK (formerly the National Asthma Campaign): www.asthma.org.uk
British Lung Foundation: www.lunguk.org
British Society for Allergy and Clinical Immunology: www.bsaci.org
British Thoracic Society: www.brit-thoracic.org.uk
General Practice Airways Group: www.gpiag.org
Global Initiative for Chronic Obstructive Pulmonary Disease: www.goldcopd.com
National Prescribing Centre: www.npc.co.uk
National Respiratory Training Centre: www.educationforhealth.org.uk
Respiratory Education and Training Centres: www.respiratoryetc.com

Guidelines

British Thoracic Society Recommendations, British Thoracic Society Standards of Care Committee. *Managing Passengers with Respiratory Disease Planning Air Travel.* 2004 http://www.brit-thoracic.org.uk/c2/uploads/FlightRevision04.pdf

British Thoracic Society/Scottish Intercollegiate Guidelines Network. British guideline on the management of asthma. *Thorax* 2003; 58 (Suppl I) S1–S94. Revised edition. November 2005, http://www.enterpriseportal2.co.uk/filestore/bts/asthmaupdatenov05.pdf

British Thoracic Society Standards of Care Subcommittee on Pulmonary Rehabilitation. BTS Statement: Pulmonary rehabilitation. *Thorax* 2001; 56: 827–834. http://www.brit-thoracic.org.uk/c2/uploads/Pulmonaryrehab.pdf

Department of Health. *Delivering investment in general practice – implementing the new GMS contract.* January, 2004. www.dh.gov.uk/assetRoot/04/07/02/31/04070231.pdf

Department of Health. *Investing in General Practice. New General Medical Services Contract.* www.dh.gov.uk/assetRoot/04/03/49/33/04034933.pdf

Department of Health. *New General Medical Services Contract Quality Indicators.* www.dh.gov.uk/assetRoot/04/05/02/53/04050253.pdf, p12.

National Institute for Clinical Excellence. *Guidance on the use of inhaler systems (devices) in children under the age of 5 years with chronic asthma.* August, 2000. www.nice.org.uk/pdf/niceINHALERguidance.pdf

National Institute for Clinical Excellence. *Inhaler devices for routine treatment of chronic asthma in older children (aged 5–15 years).* March, 2002. www.nice.org.uk/pdf/Niceinhalers_ldC38GUIDA.pdf

RPSGB Respiratory Disease Task Force. *Practice guidance on the care of people with asthma and chronic obstructive pulmonary disease*. September 2000. www.rpsgb.org/pdfs/asthmaguid.pdf

Ward MJ. Nebulisers for asthma. *Thorax* 1997; 52 (Suppl 2): S45–S48. http://www.brit-thoracic.org.uk/c2/uploads/Nebulisersforasthma.pdf

West R, McNeill A, Raw M. Smoking cessation guidelines for health professionals. A guide to effective smoking cessation interventions for the health care system. *Thorax* 1998; 53: (Suppl 5, Part 1), S1–S19. http://thorax.bmjjournals.com/cgi/reprint/53/suppl_5/S1.pdf

West R, McNeill A, Raw M. Smoking cessation guidelines for health professionals: an update. *Thorax* 2000; 55: 987–999. http://thorax.bmjjournals.com/cgi/content/full/55/12/987

Books

Holgate ST, Boushey H, Pauwels R. *Difficult Asthma*. London: Taylor and Francis, 1999.

Levy M, Hilton S. *Asthma in Practice* (Clinical Series). London: Royal College of General Practitioners, 1999.

Li JT, ed. *Pharmacotherapy of Asthma*. New York: Taylor and Francis, 2005.

National Asthma and Respiratory Training Centre (NARTC) *Simply Asthma – a Practical Pocket Book*. Cookham, Berkshire: Direct Publishing Solutions, 2002.

Price DB, Freeman D, Foster J, Scullion J. *Asthma and COPD* (In Clinical Practice Series). London: Churchill Livingstone, 2003.

Rees J, Kanabar D. *ABC of Asthma*. London: BMJ Books, 2005.

Index